NUAT BORAN THAI

Traditional Thai Medical Massage

The Nuad Boran,
Old Medicine Hospital Style

of

Northern Style Traditional Thai Yoga Therapy

By

Anthony B. James DNM, ND(T), MD(AM)

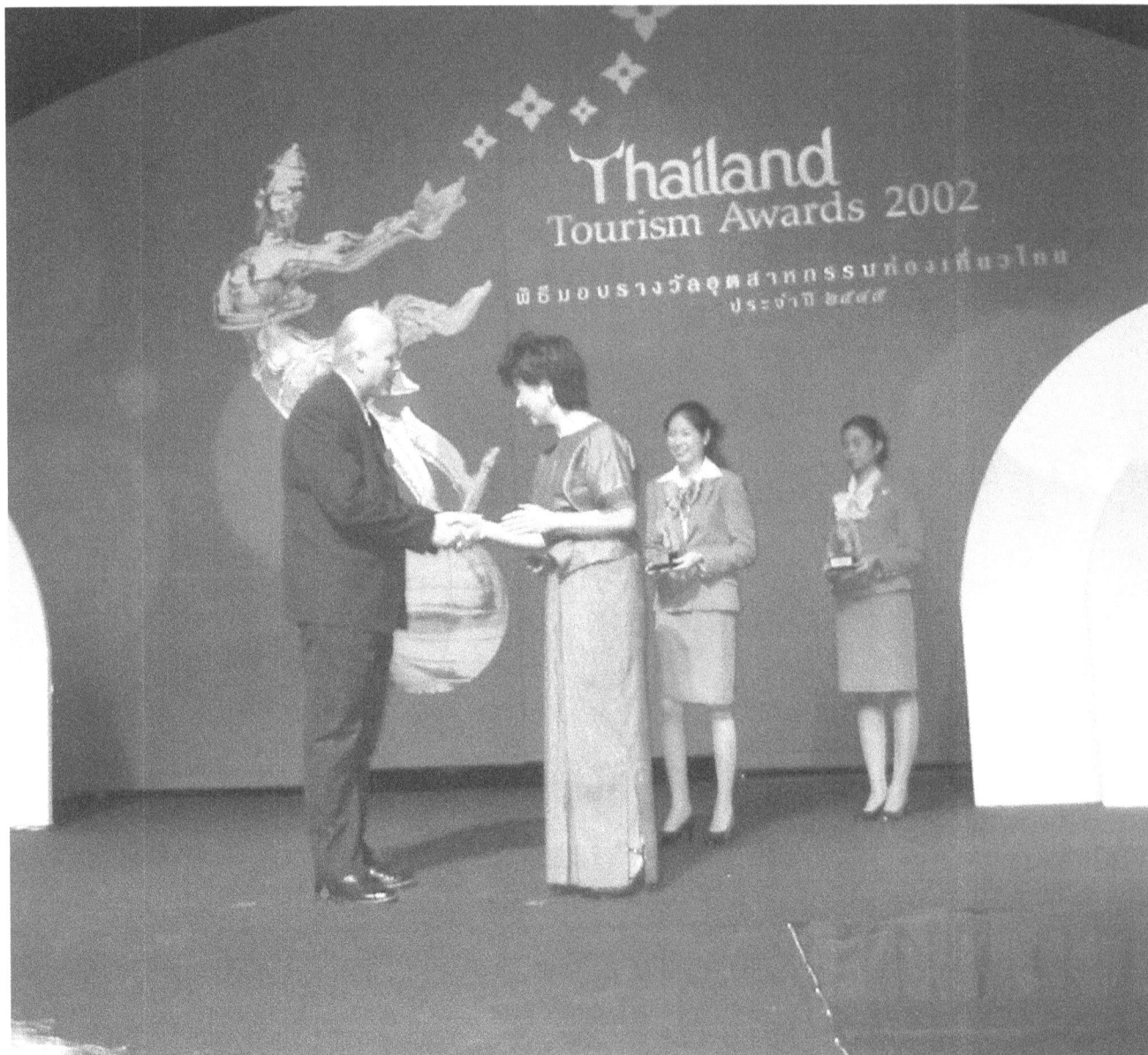

Dr. Anthony James DNM, ND(T), MD(AM), PhD, RAAP receives the prestigious "Friend of Thailand Award" from the Director General of the Tourism Authority of Thailand. The award was made in recognition for his efforts in teaching and promoting Traditional Thai Medical Massage and Nuad Boran in both Thailand and in the west. Aachan (Master Instructor) James is the first "Falang" or "Non-Thai" to receive this award for Indigenous Traditional Thai Massage (Indigenous Traditional Thai Ayurveda and Yoga Therapy).

NUAT BORAN THAI

Traditional Thai Medical Massage

The Indigenous Nuad Boran,
Old Medicine Hospital Style

of

Northern Style Traditional Thai Yoga Therapy

By

Anthony B. James DNM, ND(T), MD(AM)

NUAT BORAN THAI: Traditional Thai Medical Massage
The Indigenous Nuad Boran,Old Medicine Hospital Style

Published by
Meta Journal Press, NAIC Inc.
First Edition 1993
Second Edition 2006, 3rd. Printing
Copyright © 1993, 2018 by Anthony B. James

Printed in the U.S.A
Original art and photography Anthony B. James

Additional typography by Anthony B. James

Library of Congress: ISBN 1-886338-18-3

Please note that the author and publisher of this instructional book
is not responsible in any way whatsoever for any and all injuries which
might occur by reading and / or following the instructions herein. It is
essential that before following any of the activities, herein described,
the reader should first consult his or her physician for advise as to
whether or not to participate in the regimens described herein. This
material is presented for educational purposes only and is no substitute
for competent personal instruction.

ISBN-13: 9781886338180
51795

9 781886 338180

Dedication

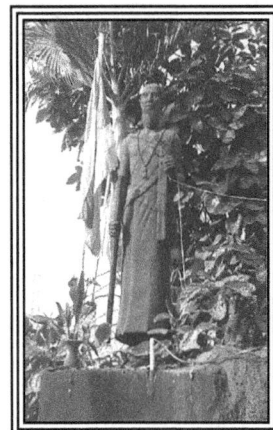

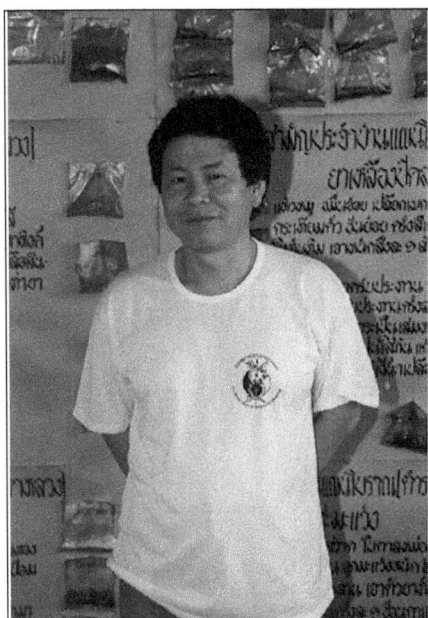

Khruu John Chongkol Setthakorn

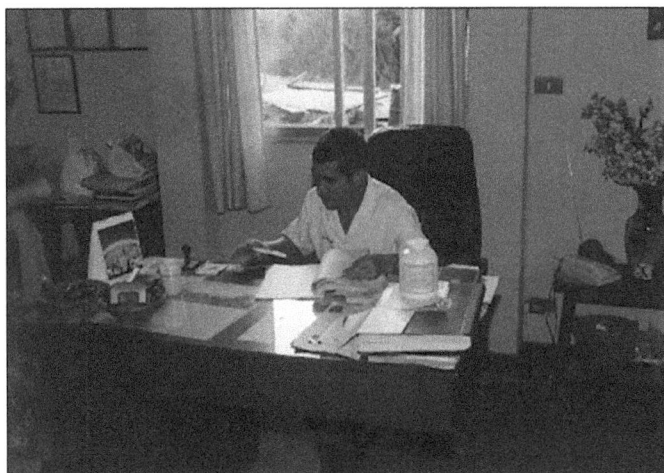

Aachan Khruu Sintorn Chaichagun

Contents

The Northern Style Wai Khruu

OM NAMO SHIVAGO SILASA A HANG KALUNIKO SAPASATANANG OSATHA TIPA-MANTANG PAPASO SURIYA-JANTANG GOMALAPATO PAKA-SESI WANTAMI BANTITO SUMET HASSO ALOKHA SUMANA-HOMI (3 times)

We invite the spirit of our founder, the father doctor Shivago, who comes to us through his saintly life. Please bring to us the knowledge of all nature, that this prayer will show us the true medicine of the universe. In the name of this mantra, we respect your help and pray that through our bodies you will bring wholeness and health to the body of our client.

PIYO-TEWA MANUSSANANG PIYO-POMA NAMUTTAMO PIYO-NAKHA SUPANANANG PINISIANG NAMA-MIHANG NAMO-PUTTAYA NAVON-NAVIEN NASATIT-NASATIEN EHI-MAMA NAVIEN-NAWE NAPAI-TANG-VIEN NAVIEN-MAHAKU EHI-MAMA PIYONG-MAMA NAMO-PUTTAYA (1 time)

The Goddess of Healing dwells in the heavens high, while mankind dwells in the world below. In the name of the founder may the heavens be reflected in the earth below so that this healing medicine may encircle the world.

NA-A NA-WA LOKHA PAYATI VINA-SANTI (3 times)

We pray for the one whom we touch, that he will be happy and that any illness will be released from him.

Thailand

Thailand is situated in the southeast part of Asia between 5 degrees
north parallel, and 21 degrees north parallel, 97 degrees east latitude
and 106 degrees longitude. It is bordered by the countries of Burma,
Campochia, Laos and Malaysia.

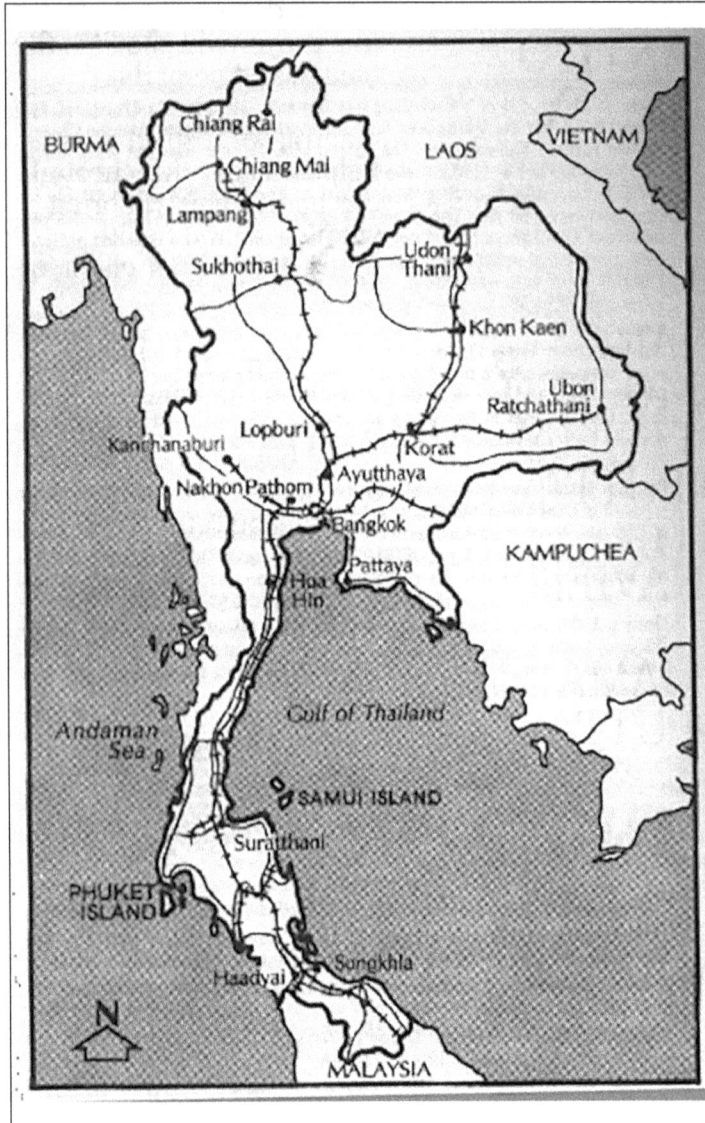

Unique Characteristics of Nuat Boran Thai

1. **No restriction of age:** Nuat Boran can be practiced on anyone of any age; the very young or the aged with great benefit. It will tonify and strengthen the young and will facilitate wellness in mind, spirit, emotions and the physical body. It will add luster, vitality to the older clients, combating the degenerative effects of aging.

2. **Nuat Boran treats total person:** The practitioner is trained to look at the person being cared for in a holistic fashion, taking into effect the ramifications of energy such as Dosha, Chakra, Sen and Mara as well as the deteriorating effects of negative emotions and energy blockages, illness or injury on many aspects of the persons body, mind, emotions and spirit.

3. **Evaluation, Assessment and therapy are combined:** Every Thai Yoga session gives the practitioner pertinent and valuable information and insight on facilitating a return to a harmonious condition. As the practitioner skillfully detects abnormalities or imbalances in the client, They are led at once to the proper method of treatment based on traditional Vedic and holistic protocals.

4. **Nuat Boran uses no mechanical devices:** Thai Yoga practitioners use the whole person to treat the whole person.

5. **No side effects:** As the specific treatment modalities used are selected on the basis of their appropriateness for the individual client, and that they are the least invasive, most natural and suitable at the time, there are no unpleasant after effects such as excessive muscular soreness.

6. .**Nuat Boran facilitates health maintenance:** Regular sessions complement other health practices by balancing all the persons energies, supporting their mental, emotional and spiritual well being, maintaining flexibility, helping eliminate waste toxins from joints and soft tissue and aiding in reducing the effects of stress and fatigue by doing all the above and relaxing the body.

7. **Nuat Boran is a balanced blending of Ayurvedic medicine, Chinese medicine and Western Holistic and Traditional Naturopathy:** This allows the practitioner greater flexibility and diversity in facilitating wellness, balance and a happy, healthy life for themselves and the client.

8. **Nuat Boran Thai emphasizes that the spiritual development of the practitioner is as important as the therapy itself.·**

9. **Nuat Boran demonstrates Promwihan Sii, or the four states of mind:** loving kindness, compassion, vicarious joy and equanimity.

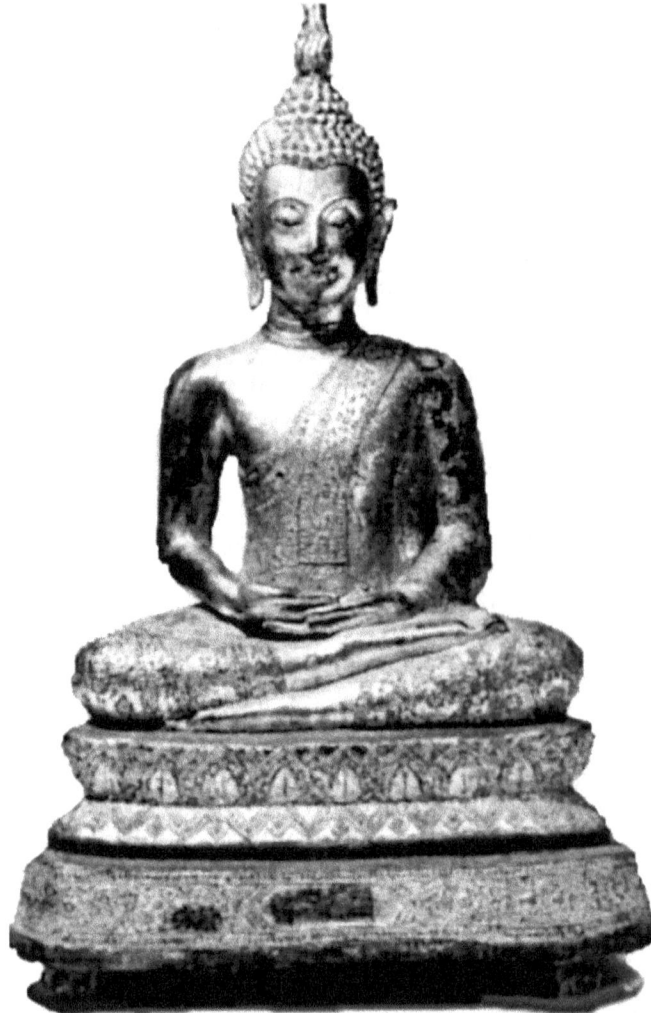

"Man must himself by his resolute efforts rise and make his way to the portals that give upon Liberty, and it is always at every moment in his power so to do. Neither are those portals locked and the key in possession of someone else from whom it must be obtained by prayer and entreaty. The door is free of all bolts and bars save those that man himself has made."

The Buddha
A Living Message
Piyadassi Thera

Chapter One: History of Nuat Thai Yoga/ Thai Massage

Thai medical massage, also called "Nuad phaen boran" or Nuat Thai, is born of a long tradition. This unique system of bodywork therapy has been taught and practiced in various locations in Thailand for about 2,500 years. The initial credit for Thai massage is actually given to one individual—a famous Indian doctor called Shivago Komalaboat. Dr. Shivago was known to be a contemporary of the Buddha and was a personal physician to Bimbisara, the Magadha king, of that period. Shivago was generally known as a close friend and personal physician to the Sangha—the order of Buddhist monks and nuns. His name is mentioned in the traditional pali canon or writings of Theravada (Hiniyama) Buddhism, and variations of this massage are practiced in Sri Lanka, Burma, Laos, Cambodia and, of course, Thailand. There is also a dramatic similarity to Amma and Tuina of China and Anma/Shiatsu of Japan.

The Wai khruu, or paying of respect, is still done partly in remembrance of his contribution to the present-day art. It is impossible to say to what extent other styles of medicine and massage have contributed to Nuat Thai's development. There is no clear written documentation of the development of the style. Primarily it has been passed from one generation to the next in the form of an oral tradition, whereby one would serve a sort of apprenticeship under a teacher, often for several years before practicing as a therapist. In general, the teachings were preserved and cherished by the monks and nuns of the Buddhist Temples. In Thailand's past, the people came to the temples for just about everything—from medical help to education. Anyone could come to the temple for food, shelter, medical or spiritual healing. Nuat Thai contributed to the emotional physical and spiritual well-being of the ancient Thais, and it continues to do so today.

In more recent times, His Majesty King Rama III engraved stone tablets duplicating those recovered from the ruins of Wat Chetaphon in the original capital, Ayudhuya. The capital was destroyed in 1767 by Burmese invaders, and fragments of the original documents were used by King Rama to make the new ones. The King installed them at Wat (Chetaphon) Pho in Bangkok. These tablets are a text of the theory behind Nuat Thai and show the Sen or lines of energy running through the body.

These charts of stone depict sixty figures, thirty of the front

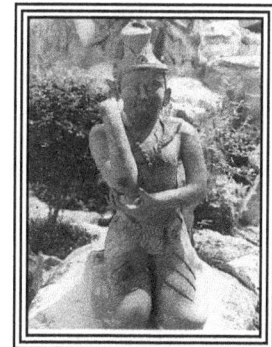
Thai Medical Massage and or Thai Massage are both slan terms for Thai Yoga.

Technically, when we originally translated the original name for laying on of hands healing as part of Classical Thai Ayurveda we used the term "Massage" as it was simply the easiest way to explain hands on healing Thai style without the spiritual context and having to explain the roles of both Thai Ayurveda and Thai Buddism.

In the last few years the term "Massage" and or "Massage Therapy" have become legislatively contentious due to the Massage Therapy and State taxation monopolies attempts to control the use of these words.

Therefore we use, emphasize and choose to use more accurate terms to describthis art to avoid confusion. Thai Yoga and Thai Ayurveda, Thai Nuad etc. are more accurate and more clearly reflect that Thai Yoga is in fact based on ancient Ayurveda Yoga and Theraveda Buddhist healing understandings and science and are unrelated entirely to what is currently being described and marketed for legal purposes as Massage or Massage Therapy.

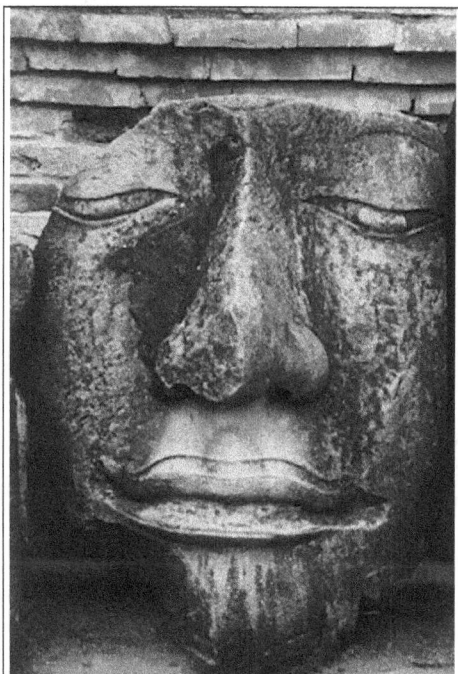
Head Section of Ancient Buddha, Ayudhya

and thirty of the back. There are channels and points clearly displayed. One interesting observation is apparent: many channels directly correspond to Chinese meridians and special or extraordinary vessels. Others correspond to the concepts of Nadis from Indian Ayruvedic medical science. The charts detail many major and minor Chakras or centers of energy.

Thai culture as a whole is a blending of many cultures from east to west (India to China), and Nuat Thai appears to demonstrate this as well. In the present day, there are two primary schools of traditional Thai medical massage and several minor, as well as many private teachers and monks or nuns who are very knowledgeable. The two primary schools are the Traditional College of Medicine, Wat Pho, Bangkok; and the Foundation of Shivago Komarpaj, Buntautuk Old Medical Hospital in Chiang Mai. Traditional Thai massage is also taught in many local temples and by various competent individuals from Chiang Mai to Sri Lanka, as well as in sword-fighting schools such as the Krabi Krabong of The Buddhai/ Swan Institute in Nongkam.

Origins of The Thai People
Thai historians estimate that the original home or place of origin of the Thai people is in the north of what we today call Siberia. In a latter period, these people immigrated in a southerly direction and eventually settled in China in an area from the Huang Ho River downward. About 2,500 years before the Buddhist Era, Chinese people displaced from their part of the land crossed the Thien Charn Mountain and began to infiltrate the basin of the Huang Ho River. They met the "Ai Lao" or "Thai" people there. The Chinese called these people "Tai," meaning powerful and prosperous.

Eventually, there was competition between the Chinese and the Thais, with the Thais being greatly outnumbered. They were compelled to withdraw in a southerly direction.

The Thai united and set up a large territory which they called "Narn Chao." They controlled this area from approximately B.E. 1192 to B.E. 1797, for a total of about 600 years. The Chinese continued to press the Thai people until finally a famous Chinese emperor, Nquan Lee Cho or Kubla Khan, led a huge army against the Narn Chao and conquered the territory. Most of the Thais fled further south, although there are still ethnic Thai people in the area of Yunan China today. The remaining Thai people settled in the area in which they now predominate, and set up independent kingdoms much like those of India of the same period. These kingdoms were assimilated into the kingdom of Ayudhya around B.E. 1913.

Krungthep Dvaravati Sri Ayudhya
Krungthep Dvaravati Sri Ayudhya was Capital of Thailand for 417 years under 33 kings of the Ayudhya Dynasty. At its peak, this Capital was larger and cleaner than contemporary European capitals. Ayudhya was founded on an island bordered by the Lopburi River on

the North, the Pasak River on the East, and the Chao Phyra River to the West and South.

In the 11th century A.D., before the Thais settled, there existed a small outpost settlement formed and named Ayudhya by the Khmers, who dominated this region of the Menam Chao Phrya. Ayudhya was of some importance because it formed a boundary with the U-Thong (a vassal State under the Sukho Thai — the first integrated Thai kingdom, called the "Cradle of Thai Civilization"). The first King of Ayudhya was Somdej Phra Ramathibodi. The kingdom was ruled in succession by 33 kings for 417 years, from A.D. 1350 to A.D. 1767.

When the original buildings of the new capital were completed in A.D. 1353, King Ramathibodi built Wat Buddhai/Swan on the site of his first residence at Wienglak. It is this wat or temple which became the home and training ground for the Kabri-Kabrong Fighting Arts. These Arts were practiced by the monks as a form of meditation and physical exercise, and the monks themselves were responsible for training the royal family and the military. Essentially, this tradition continues to the present day. Similarly, Wat Chetaphon (Wat Pho) was also established a teaching center for traditional healing and medicinal arts.

The period of settlement in the old Capital of Ayudhya is significant in that it was marked with numerous altercations and battles with the neighboring country of Burma.

The Burmese captured the Capital of Siam (as it was called in B.E. 2112), and took most of the population back to Burma as prisoners. For a time, Siam was a vassal State of the Burmese.

Around B.E. 2126, the Thais, led by the self-declared Thai King Narasuan, revolted against the Burmese. King Narasuan had become famous for being a great boxer or fighter of Buddha Swan. King Narasuan and the Burmese Crown Prince met in single combat, mounted on elephants. They dueled fiercely, and King Narasuan defeated the Prince and the Burmese army was routed.

Sometime later, around B.E. 2325, King Pra Buddha Yod Fa Chula Loke ascended the throne as the first King of the Chakri Dynasty. Thailand continued as an independent State from this time to the present day, where it is currently under the patronage of H.M. King Phumibol Adul Yadej, ninth King of the Chakri Dynasty. The capital of Thailand in the present time is Krungthep, or Bangkok; where the King resides in the Grand Palace next to Wat Phra Kao, the Temple of the Emerald Buddha; and Wat Pho, the Temple of the Reclining Buddha.

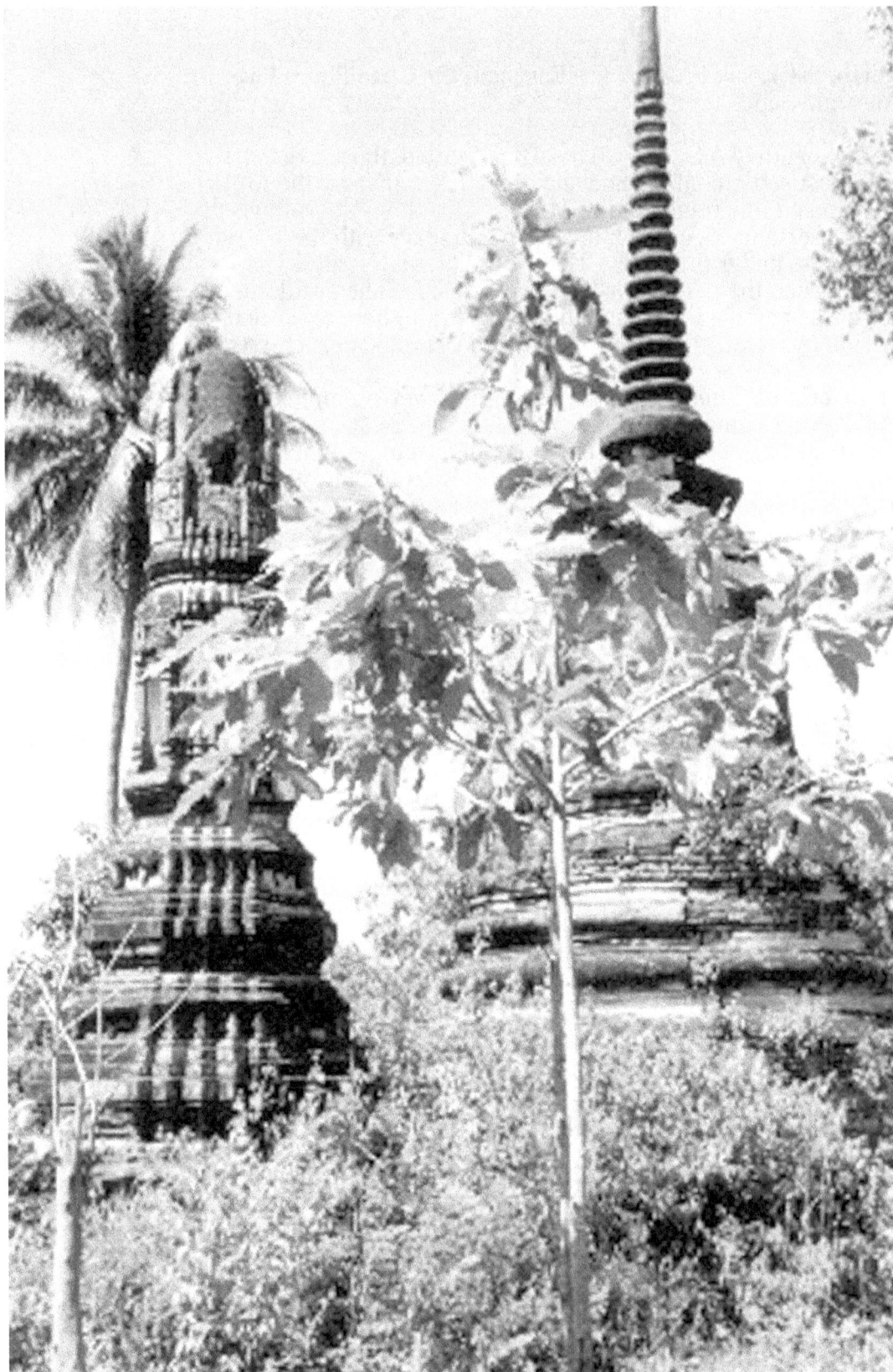

The original and sacred medical texts have been stored for centuries in Chedi like these, found in Ayudthaya province.

How To Study Thai Massage

Nuat Thai is a highly sophisticated and well-developed form of healing and manipulative therapy. Refined by diligent practitioners over a period of thousands of years, Nuat Thai is not an anachronism, but a valid and scientifically-based form of health care with limitless possibilities. These possibilities are limited only by the technical sophistication and imagination of the practitioner. The Thais believe all things should be considered with an open mind. This book should serve to give a very good idea as to the variety of benefits realistically attainable through the practice of Nuat Thai. However, no book is an adequate substitute for a competent instructor or school. It is important to place a priority on finding a personal teacher, if you really wish to master this or any sophisticated form of health care management. There are nuances of technique and application which cannot adequately be conveyed, however detailed the text or photographs. If you choose to undertake to practice, work with a reliable, consistent partner. GO SLOW! It is especially well-integrated with other energy, or spiritually based Oriental systems such as Reiki, Shiatsu, AMMA, Tui-Na or Jin Shin Do. Although this system is not "Massage" or "Massage Therapy" as legally described in most state laws, this system may also be used quite successfully in cooperation with many Western methods, such as massage and or massage therapy variations.

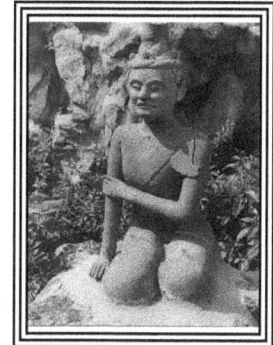

The following principles, taught to me by friend and former teacher Sifu Dan Inosanto, will serve you, the student, as they have served me.

- **Research your own experience**

- **Absorb what is useful**

- **Reject what is useless**

- **Add something specifically your own**

To "research your own experience" is to take stock of your capabilities physically, emotionally and spiritually before you ask for more. Find that which is relevant and useful from your own life and experience. Find that which is not useful. Correctly appraising one's skill or knowledge often becomes the beginning of attaining wisdom.

To "absorb what is useful" is to consciously expose oneself to experience and information which is expected to increase one's being. Knowledge may be useful; practical experience may be useful. But it is not enough just to gain access or proximity to those things which are useful—one must be prepared to receive them, to take them in. Zen practitioners have a saying: "One may not add to a full cup." Empty your cup!

To "reject what is useless" is to purposefully remove unproductive elements from your life, or to extricate yourself from an unproductive area or situation. It also has the connotation of giving up or releasing attitudes and emotional baggage which may buffer or hinder you from reaching your true potential. There is an element of being selective of the many impressions chosen to be a part of one's life. It also refers to "doing," to being an active participant, an "author of your own experience."

To "add something specifically your own" is to draw upon your personal nature, experience and background. Your intuitions, insights, skills and information are as real, valid, and as valuable as those from any other source. Your intuition may be correct. You may very well know what to do or where to go. This "adding to" is what makes the teaching personal and really practical. What you will end up with is a science and art that is practical, powerful and uniquely personal.

Additionally, the following tips will be of use.

1. When working with the body, everything is important; nothing is insignificant. Seek to see the big picture by seeing the whole person, mind, body and spirit.

2. Don't just go through the motions. Try to understand why things are done as they are.

3. Don't do anything to anyone until or unless you know the reason, and know what to expect as a likely result of your actions and intent.

4. Intent is more valuable than technique. There may be many ways to accomplish the objective, but first you must be clear as to what that objective is. Additionally, focused intent affects energy.

5. Seek to master the technical aspects of the work; the pathways and SEN, the physiology and philosophy of the art as presented. Develop a clear understanding of the Western anatomy and physiology; know the muscles, bones, nerves and circulatory systems affected by each movement.

6. You should be able to trace the SEN in the body, and readily locate the chakras and major energy points.

7. The therapist's own strength and flexibility are important. Tai Chi, Chi Gung and Yoga training are all valuable and productive. Internal training and meditation are great assets: how can you direct an influence another's energy with sensitivity, if you have no valid concept of your own?

8. Phaa Khruu said, "Go slow, slow. The slow, slow way is best." Wait for the response to happen—everything in life changes at its own rate or in its own time.

9. Repeat and repeat every movement until the technique and method

become second nature. Relax and train until you are able to function

instinctively; at this point you will be able to bring your full attention to the client, as opposed to thinking about what to do next.

10. Follow the Taoist maxim, "At least do no harm."

Purposes of Thai Yoga, Thai Massage

Thai Yoga is used to facilitate and promote a harmonious state of being. The ancient Thai people recorded various states of disease and imbalance within the body, the mind and the emotions. Over a period of time, they carefully devised creative and practical methods of influencing the course of balances in every part of a persons life. This was important, as imbalances prevented people from fully experiencing life in a productive way. If someone suffered a trauma or injury, then laying on of hands was the primary method or vehicle of rehabilitation. If, for instance, a person suffered from disease related to poor circulation, it was noticed that praying and laying hands on the affected person could not only reduce the swelling, it could reduce or diminish the pain and emotional trauma as well. Thai Yoga could expand a person's ability to move, or relax someone overly excited.

Over the years, the list of benefits of Thai Yoga has expanded but these can be categorized generally as :

A. Relaxation
B. Reduction of pain
C. Reduction of swelling/edema
D. Increased range of motion
E. Management of stress
F. Passive exercise
G. Enhanced body/mind connection
H. Evaluation of soft-tissue status
I. Preparation for exercise
J. Detoxification of soft tissue
K. Expression of loving, kindness or nurturing
L. Maintenance of general health without indications of disease
M. Reduction of Negative Emotional Patterns
N. Balance of energy within Chakra, Prana Nadi or Sen, Marma and
     Wind Gates.

Traditionally, the Thai have always considered therapeutic Yoga as a vital and integral part of their health maintenance practices. Until relatively recently (World War I), the use of Yoga Ayurveda and Yoga therapy and the use of herbal preparations constituted the bulk of their formal medical treatment for all diseases. Even with the advent of modern Western-style hospitals and medical-delivery models, the Thai people continue to rely on traditional energy and spiritually based therapeutic remedies.

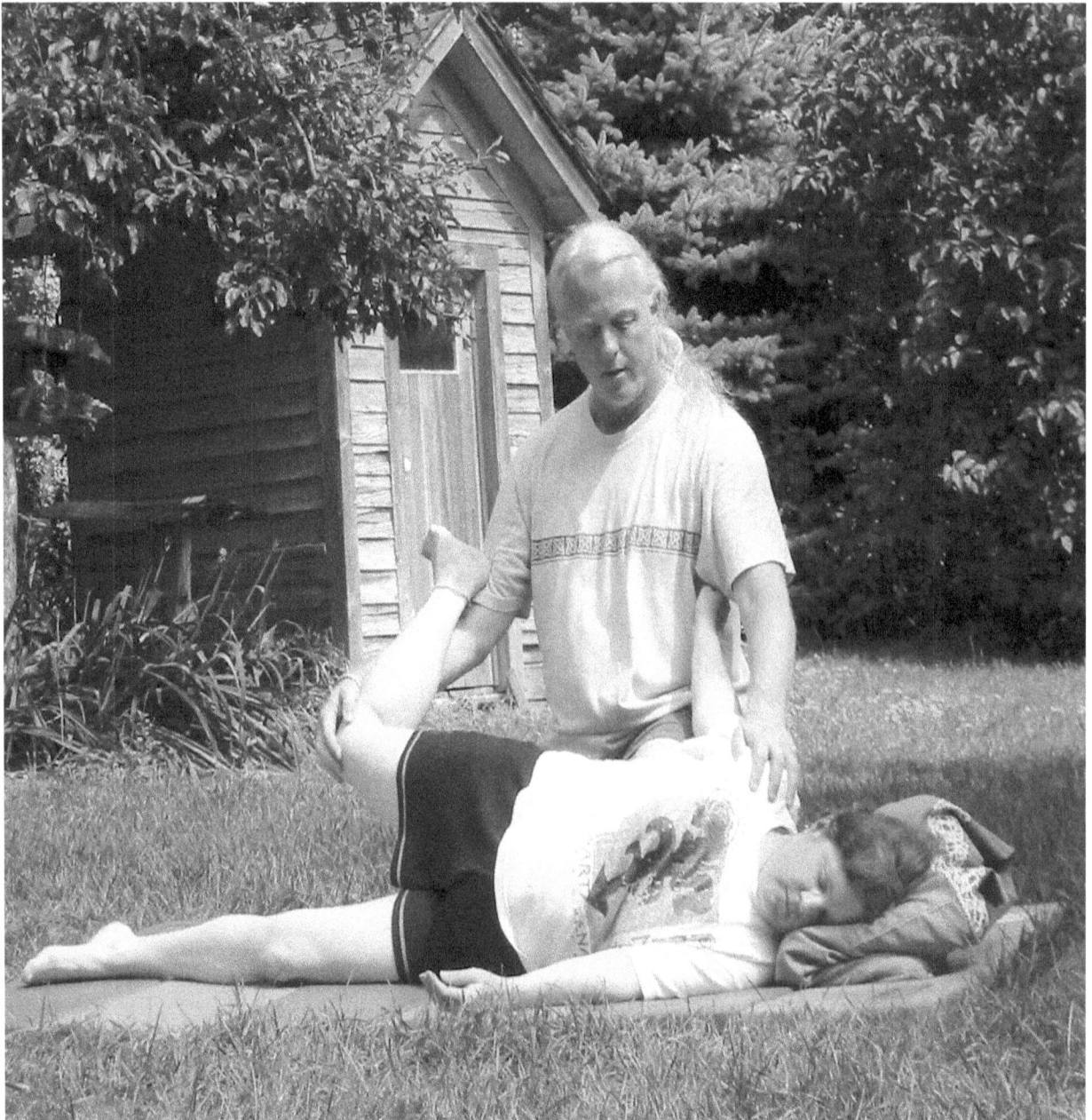

The Northern style of Nuad Boran Thai clearly shows the grace and form of all true Yoga disciplines. Aachan Anthony James demonstrates the Ardis Dhanurasana or Half Bow Pose in the Side Lying Position.

Chapter Three: Preparation for the Session

The Therapist

The therapist should be mentally, emotionally and physically ready; that is, in a frame of mind to use the massage as a means of expressing care and compassion.

The therapist should be relaxed and healthy, not unduly under stress and certainly not under the influence of drugs or alcohol. Cleanliness and hygiene are paramount. Warm hands and short finger nails are also important.

The theripist should wear loose, comfortable clothing, allowing for freedom of movement and the circulation of the therapist's own energy. It is inappropriate to wear rings, watches and bracelets which might distract or interfere with the sessions.

Before beginning, the theripist should practice the puja or prayer. It does not have to be a Buddhist prayer, as the therapist may follow any creed. But the minute of quiet meditation serves to ground one before actually touching the client.

Additionally, the clothing and dress of the therapist should be clean and neat, a reflction of the therapist's personal hygiene which shoud be exemplary. To prepare well for the intended work at hand is to be responsible for the intended results. To be ambigous inpreparation and action is to predicate ambiguous results. Everything is important. To quote the first century stoic philosopher Epictetus:
> " No part of life is exempt from needing our careful attention. Will you do anything the worse by taking pains and the better by neglect? Is any other, even the minutest operation best performed heedlessly?

The Client
The client should be ready, able and willing to receive the massage. Massage is an intimate interaction involving often intense physical contact. Thrust is imperative.
The client should undress only to his or her level of comfort, not for the convenience or comfort of the therapist. Nuat Thai may be performed perfectly with clothing on. If the client is clothed, the clothing should be light and unrestrictive to allow for unhindered movements. Tight undergarments and jewelry should be removed.

The client should be on a thick blanket, futon or mat. The surface should not be too soft, as a soft surface tends to absorb the pressure the therapist is trying to generate.

The Corpse Pose (Savasana)
The therapist begins the therapy by placing the client supine in the corpse pose, or savasana. The client is instructed and assisted into a position lying flat on the back. The body is then adjusted to relieve or release any unnecessary tension. This is done by gently rocking the

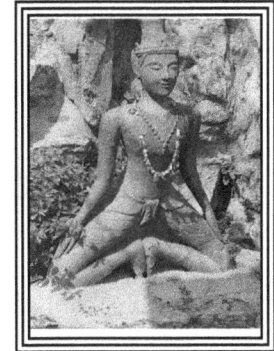

client's body, beginning at the hips and working down the legs. The legs are turned in and out several times, then allowed to fall gently to rest.

It is useful to instruct the client to tuck the chin inward slightly, elongating the neck and helping to relax the spine. The therapist may roll the client's head back and forth before allowing it to sink and settle into its natural resting position.

It is a good idea to concentrate or focus the client's attention on the breath by having him breathe deeply and slowly from the abdomen. He will experience a relaxing state and a sense of sinking into the mat.

Follow this same procedure when the client is positioned in the prone corpse position, as well.

Positioning The Client
Specific positioning of the client is addressed for each technique, but as a general rule, the client should always be comfortable and well-supported; the client should not have to exert any effort to hold himself in position.

There definitely are times when it is appropriate to use pillows and bolsters to support or brace the client securely. A good example of this might be when the client is positioned in the Side Lying Position (S.L.P.), and support is appropriate for the head.

The Setting
A comfortable and pleasing environment is complementary to a peaceful state of mind. A peaceful mind complements a harmonious physical state, both for therapist and client alike.

The optimal area for massage should be distraction-free, clean, quiet, well-ventilated. Outdoor places, such as under a shade tree or in a grassy field, on a beach, beside a pond or lake, or in a forest are all excellent choices. If the session is held in an office environment, it should be warm and comfortable, appealing and inviting. Songs or music without lyrics are preferable to enhance a relaxing mood. Many therapists may work well sharing the same pleasant space.

Pleasant aromas or natural fragrances are also complementary. In Thailand, it is common to find fresh flowers around the massage area. Incense may be used, but care should be taken to avoid over-stimulating the therapist's environment, since some clients may be sensitive to the smoke.

There should be no bright light shining directly on the client. Indirect, soft light is preferable. The exception to this is when doing very specific therapy. For example, when treating a knee or jaw injury for trigger points, specific lights may be necessary.

Principles of Nuat Thai
The therapist and client should remain "centered" throughout the session. That means mentally and physically concentrated on the present moment and movement. Partake of the experience without straying into the past or future. If thoughts which are not relevant come up, do not pursue them to excite them or give them more substance. Rather, simply let them pass on without owning or encouraging them; they will pass if you do not identify with or attach to them. It should be understood that there will be a minimum of conversation, which usually has a tendency to wander (i.e., "Who won the game Saturday?" or the like). The therapist should take a quiet moment, but it is better if the therapist and client can pray or meditate together to calm the mind. The client may be instructed to bring his attention specifically to the area of the body being treated.

Go Slow. Whenever there is the question, "Am I going too fast?" the answer usually is, "Yes." When in doubt, slow down. Phaa Kruu Kitniyom says, "The slow, slow way is the best." All pressure, regardless of how it is to be applied, is applied in a slow, firm and flowing manner. Technique should be applied by manipulating the body weight, as opposed to using hand and arm strength. Lean and shift to push and to pull.

As a general rule, most pressure is applied for five (5) seconds, and then released slowly. If a specific area is ischemic, or if it has taut bands of tissue, pressure may be held longer until the tissue releases in ten to twelve (10 to 12) seconds. Once released, move smoothly to the next point.

When applying pressure, use the breath to facilitate the flow of energy. Take a breath, and exhale slowly as you apply pressure. Visualize energy rising from the lower Dan Tien area upward, and flowing out of the arms and hands into the points of pressure. Sometimes it is useful to visualize this flow of energy as a colored light. Having a correct mental picture of the transfer of energy will intensify the results of your effort.

Often it is beneficial for the therapist to close his or her eyes, as this develops proprioceptive facilitation; that is, develops the therapist's ability to actually perceive or sense changes in tissue or energy states. Traditionally, Thai massage was especially performed by the blind. It is beneficial to instruct the client not to resist pressure. The client should "give before it" and exhale, releasing tension.

Give the client a few moments to regroup and to recover at the end of the session. This time is especially important, as all the physical and energetic changes brought on by the massage do not manifest immediately. It is not uncommon for clients to report changes over a period of days after a good session.

General Notes on Devising Treatments

A. Always work within the pain or sensitivity tolerance of the client. A good rule of thumb is to use medium to firm pressure. This pressure may described on a continuum of one to ten. One (1) represents pressure so light the client cannot tell they are being touched, and ten (10) represents pressure so excruciating they will run screaming from the room. To elicit the necessary response in the nervous system, soft tissue and fascia, the level of pressure should be about
a seven (7) or eight (8) on this scale.

B. Work or massage the SEN or the channel closest to the specific area of pain or injury. Treat the whole line.

C. Facilitate the range of motion in any joints near the area of greatest concern.

D. Treat the pressure points in proximity to the area of concern.

E. When there is more than one area of concern, prioritize them according to gravity or severity.

Note: Oftentimes, severe injuries like broken bones do not hurt as much as bad bruises or sprains.

F. Always look at the whole person before finalizing the course of treatment.

G. When a physician or doctor prescribes a particular course of treatment, follow their guidelines explicitly. Do not "wing it!"

H. Clients who do not respond to the treatment, or those whose condition worsens progressively or acutely after the treatment, should immediately be referred to a competent physician.

I. Begin with a general release, gradually become more specific or use more pressure, and finish with the general once again.

J. Pay attention to the space between one technique and another. The transition is no less important, as it may reveal much and contribute much to the work as well.

"One must not believe anything without verification, and one must not do anything until one understands why..."
P.D. Ouspensky, The Fourth Way

Principles of Treatment

The most important point is that your co-facilitating release of energy in Yoga Asana using energy, attention, consciousness, breath and pressure. Actual pressure or physical contact is incidental to sharing your love, compassion, joy and equinimity to the client. No different than giving some one a hug of brotherly or sisterly love! Our expression of brotherly love just happens to be more sophisticated than most. But the purpose for touching at all remains the same.

Make your own health and welfare a priority for your own sake, as well as an example to your client. Have regular bodywork, preferably several times a month.

All application of pressure is performed using the energy of the whole body. Don't work with hand and arm strength, but rather work from your lower chakras and Dan Tien.

Practice all the principles of proper body mechanics and keep well-balanced, distributing your weight evenly between the hands and the knees or feet.

Watch for unnecessary tension in your own body, and relax these areas as the tension appears. This will conserve your strength and keep your own energy from being restricted as you work.

Always keep both hands on the client. This is for security, balance and proper polarity, as one hand represents a positive pole and the other a negative.

As you work, maintain surveillance of the condition of the whole body, as well as the specific areas you are currently working on. Be aware and give consideration to areas of heat, cold, swellings, soft-tissue variations, taut bands, or tight or hard areas that should be soft, etc.

It is soothing and comforting both for the client and the therapist to progress with a steady rhythm. Practice your transitions from one technique to the next so that they become smooth and fluid, like a dance.

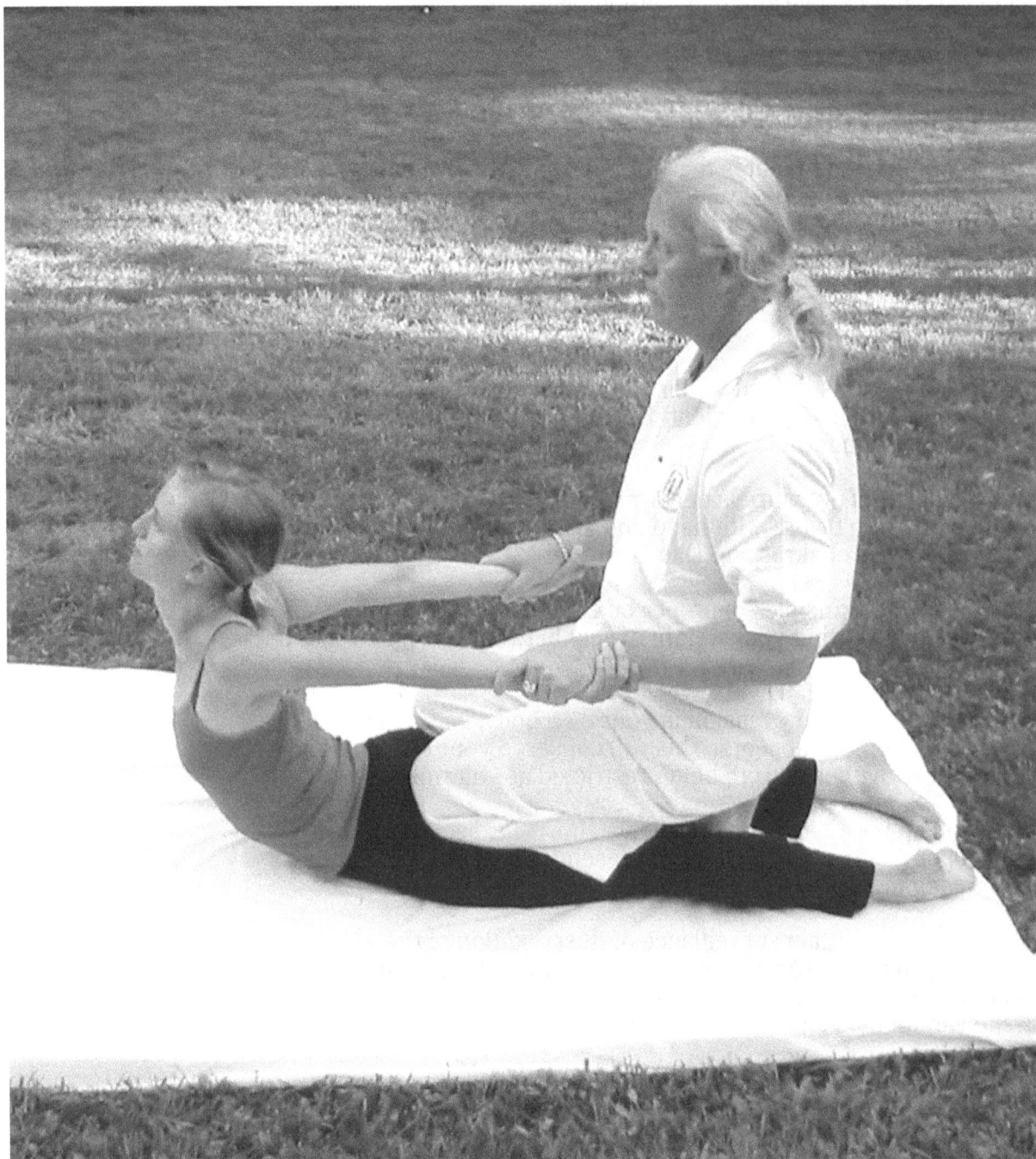

Range of motion and pressure must always be appropriate for individual client as well as the therapists at all times. Strength, balance and range of motion are always balanced with sensitivity and loving kindness.

Section One: Basic Techniques and Movements Used In Massage

1. Thumb pressure—Use the ball of the thumb to ischemically compress or to apply direct pressure. Press firmly with the pad of the thumb.

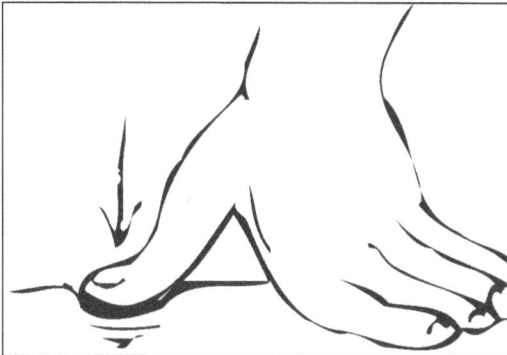

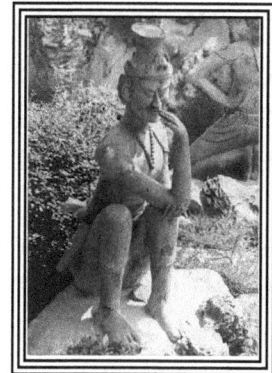

2. Reinforced thumb pressure—One thumb is placed on top of the other to provide more potential pressure and greater control than feasible with one thumb only. The reinforced thumb also reduces fatigue for the therapist.

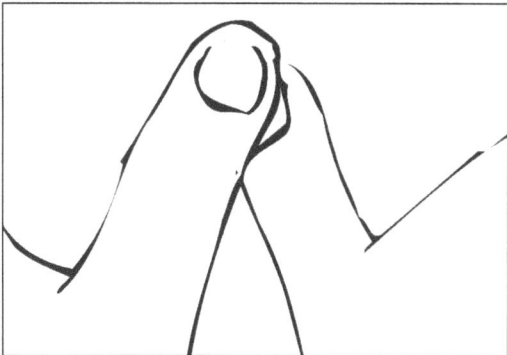

3. Circular thumb pressure—Using either one thumb or reinforced thumb pressure, describe small half-circles inward, then release out; again using pressure applied with the pad of the thumb.

4. Rotating thumbs—Using both thumbs, rotate each one in circles, either in opposition or in unison, with light pressure.

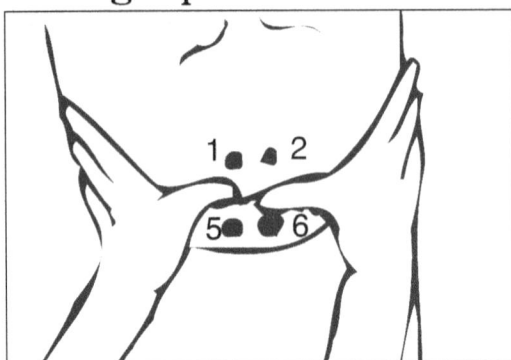

5. Thumb-walking—Exchange pressure from one thumb to the other in an alternating fashion. Lead with one hand and follow closely with the other.

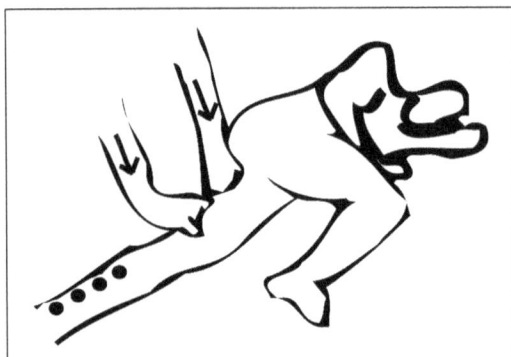

6. Rolling thumbs—Press inward with both thumbs and then rotate over or away from the therapist's body. This may also be a rotation across the fascia, muscles, Sen lines, meridians or nerves.

7. Snake thumb pressure —The thumbs undulate (Klai Sen) from side to side as the hand moves along the line.

8. Palm pressure—Keep the arms locked out, and use the shifting of the body's weight to create and apply pressure through the palms. The hands may be together or separated. This technique emphasizes a soft hand, with the fingers completely relaxe

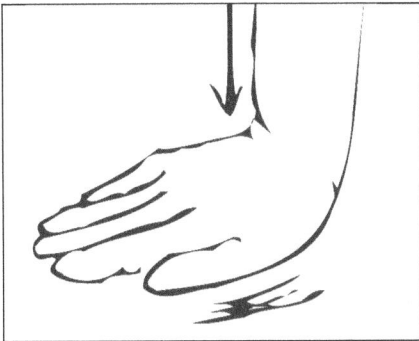

9. Palm stretching—Place the hands at the opposite ends of the body section being worked, and press outward away from each other; thus lengthening and creating a gentle traction effect.

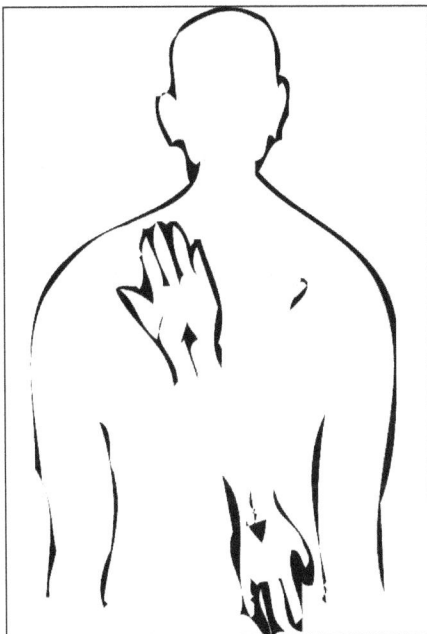

10. Palm walking—Exchange and alternate pressure from one hand to the other, moving forward and backward.

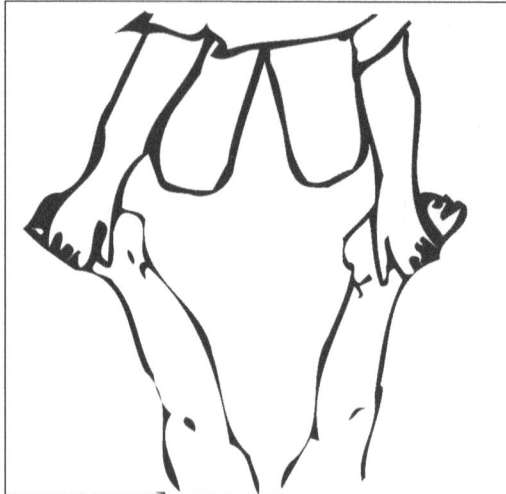

11. Circular palm pressure—The palms are pressed in either small or large circles. This is generally a technique for superficial stimulation or moving body fluids.

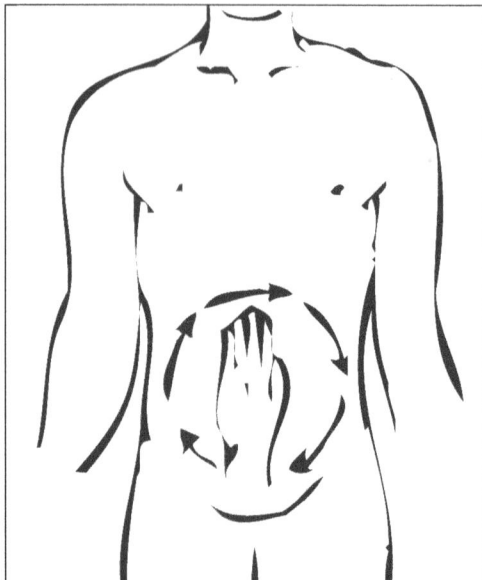

12. Rolling palms—Similar to the technique of the rolling thumbs. Press in with direct pressure, and then rotate away or across the fascia, muscle, Sen or nerve.

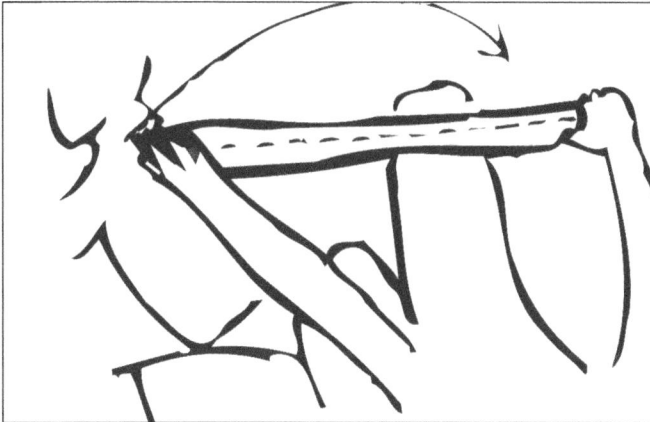

13. Elbow pressure—Use direct pressure with the point of the elbow to give more penetration in large, soft areas; or especially tough areas; than is possible with the thumbs alone.

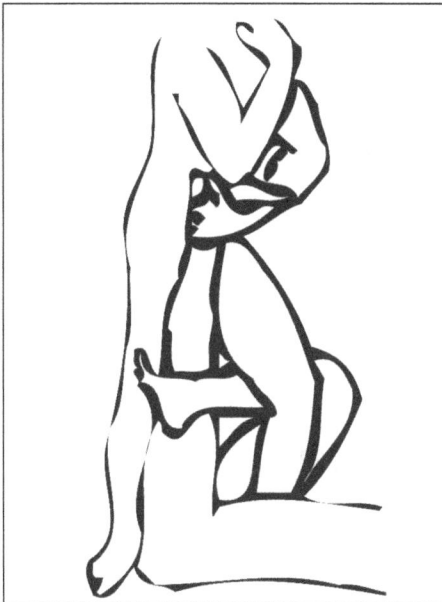

14. Forearm pressure—Used to work a broader surface than preferred with the elbow, or to work areas that are more sensitive to more specific pressure.

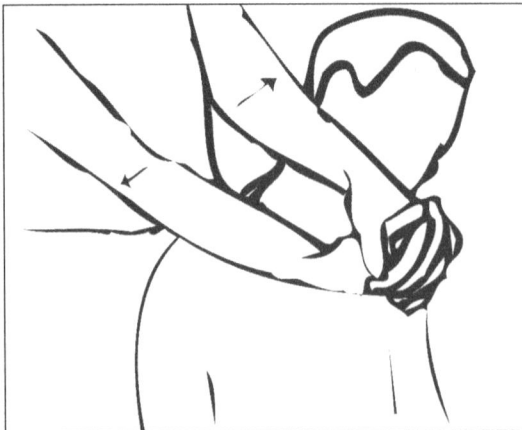

15. Circular digital pressure—The fingers of the hand are held firmly together and straight out. The tips of the fingers are the primary contact surface, and are applied in small circles.

16. Reinforced finger pressure—The stiffened, outstretched fingers of one or both hands are used to press directly on various pressure points and nerves.

17. Finger-tip brushing—Use the fingers like a brush, pulling them softly and quickly across the body. Generally finish with a sweeping motion away from or off the body.

18. Pinching and rolling—Tissue is squeezed between the thumb and fingers (especially good for toes and fingers). The tissue also may be pulled away from the body.

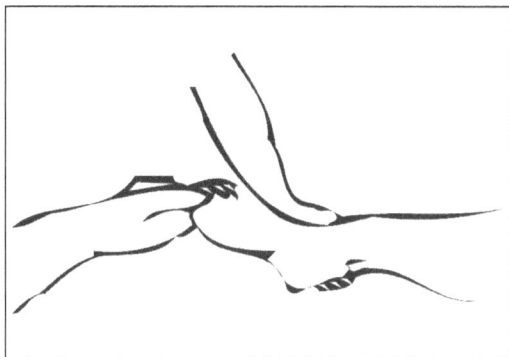

19. Hooking—With the finger bent into the shape of a hook and held rigid, pull into the area to be treated.

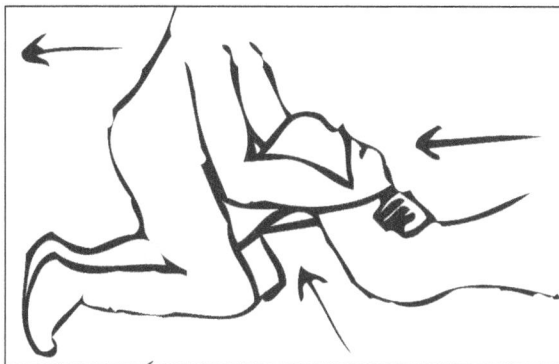

20. Walking hook—Move the hands held in the hook position back and forth along a line.

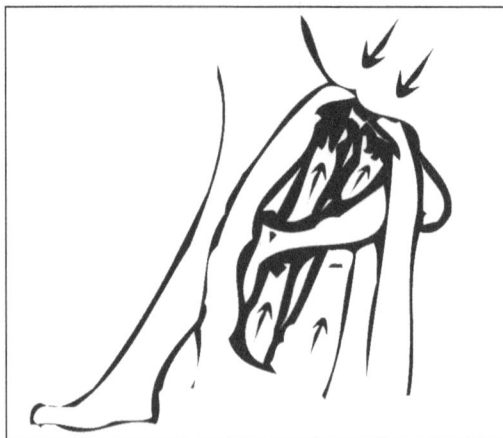

21. Vise or squeezing techniques—Interlock the fingers and squeeze the hands together by moving the elbows inward towards each other.

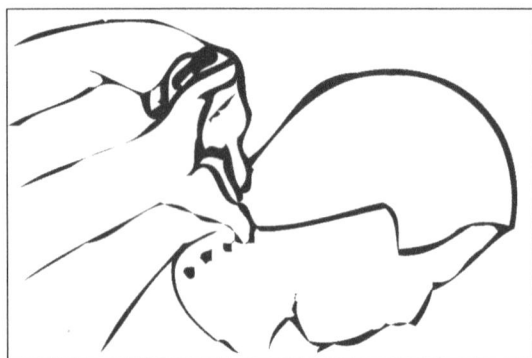

22. Tiger-hand technique—A pinching technique; squeezing points firmly between thumb and fingers, which are held firmly.

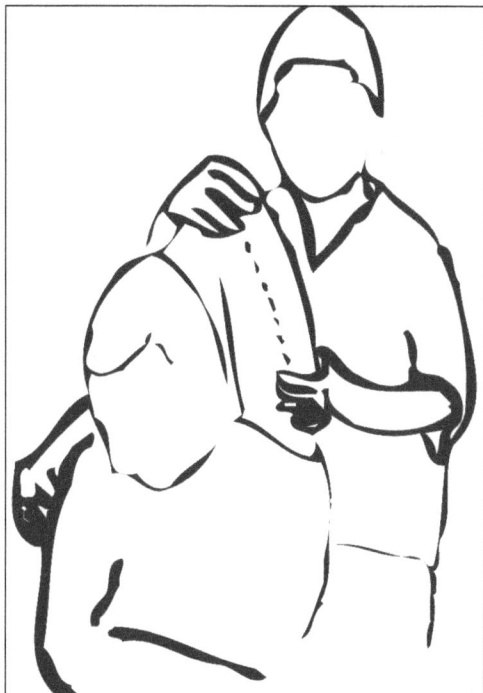

23. Kneading—Cross the soft tissue firmly between the thumb and fingers, and squeeze alternately.

24. Foot pressure—The feet are used directly to work various Sen and points. The heel is used primarily for point application, and the broad foot for more general. This even includes walking or standing on various parts of the body.

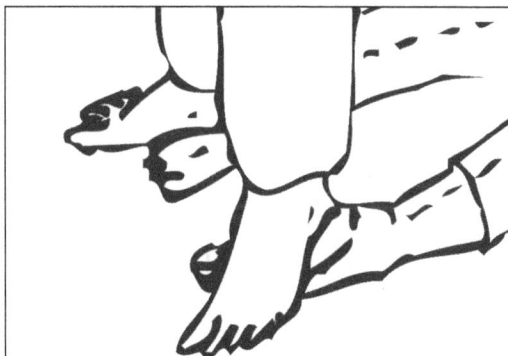

25. Hitting—Alternate open and closed-hand techniques, striking areas of the body using light to moderate pressure. Slapping-type movements may be included as well. There are fifteen or more basic striking techniques, and variations are numerous. Thai striking techniques are very similar to Chinese AMMA and Japanese Shiatsu/ANMA techniques.

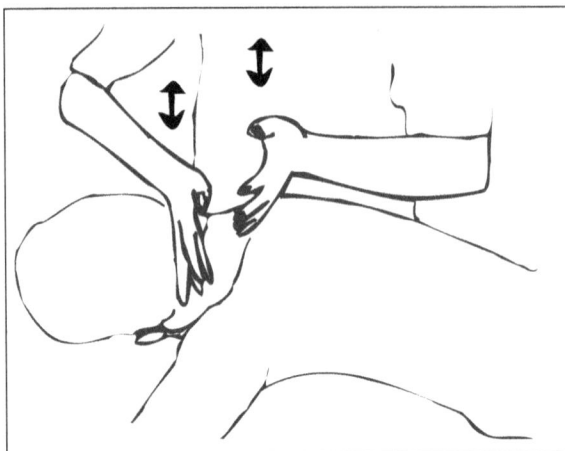

26. Knee pressure—Kneel directly on the area to be treated; allow the hands to stabilize other areas or to work conjunctive pressure points used to cover broad areas with great control.

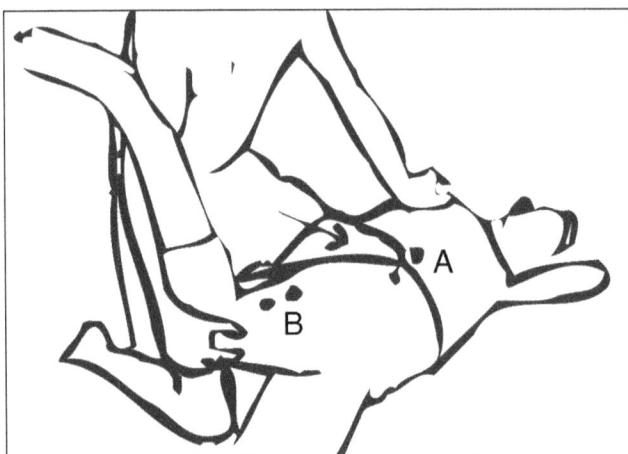

Section Two: Rocking Technique

Just as we gently and instinctively rock babies and children to calm them, we often do the same with adults. When we are holding someone who is sick, injured or otherwise disturbed, there is a natural inclination to rock that person. Generally, this has the immediate effect of calming and soothing, and it has a deep nurturing quality as well. The whole body may be rocked gently, or the therapist may rock separate body parts, such as the extremities.

Generally, rocking facilitates grounding of the client, and relaxation as well. Gently rock a leg back and forth before working the energy lines, for instance.

This simple technique, so beneficial on its own, is a good preparation for deeper work. Additionally, it is an excellent finishing technique after intense pressure or stretching. Rocking, by freeing joints and tissue to move, creates space in the body, also facilitating the flow of energy.

Section Three: Body Mechanics

Principles of proper and correct posture and economy of movement should be adhered to at all times. There is always a more efficient way to perform a given technique.

Avoid positions which strain the operator or which seem precarious. Always sit, stand or kneel close to the client to bring your center of gravity to bear. Keep the weight of your body evenly distributed in order to reduce fatigue. When using the hands, the knees or the elbows, share the load with the parts of your body not directly involved.

For instance, when applying pressure with the palms, distribute your weight between the knees and the hands. Keep your back straight and chin elevated. Most of all, relax and breathe. When you notice that you are straining, release the tension in that area and adjust to a better position.

With time and experience, your body will hunt for the path of least resistance. Proper and efficient body posture and body mechanics is one of the keys to maintaining and developing tactile sensitivity.

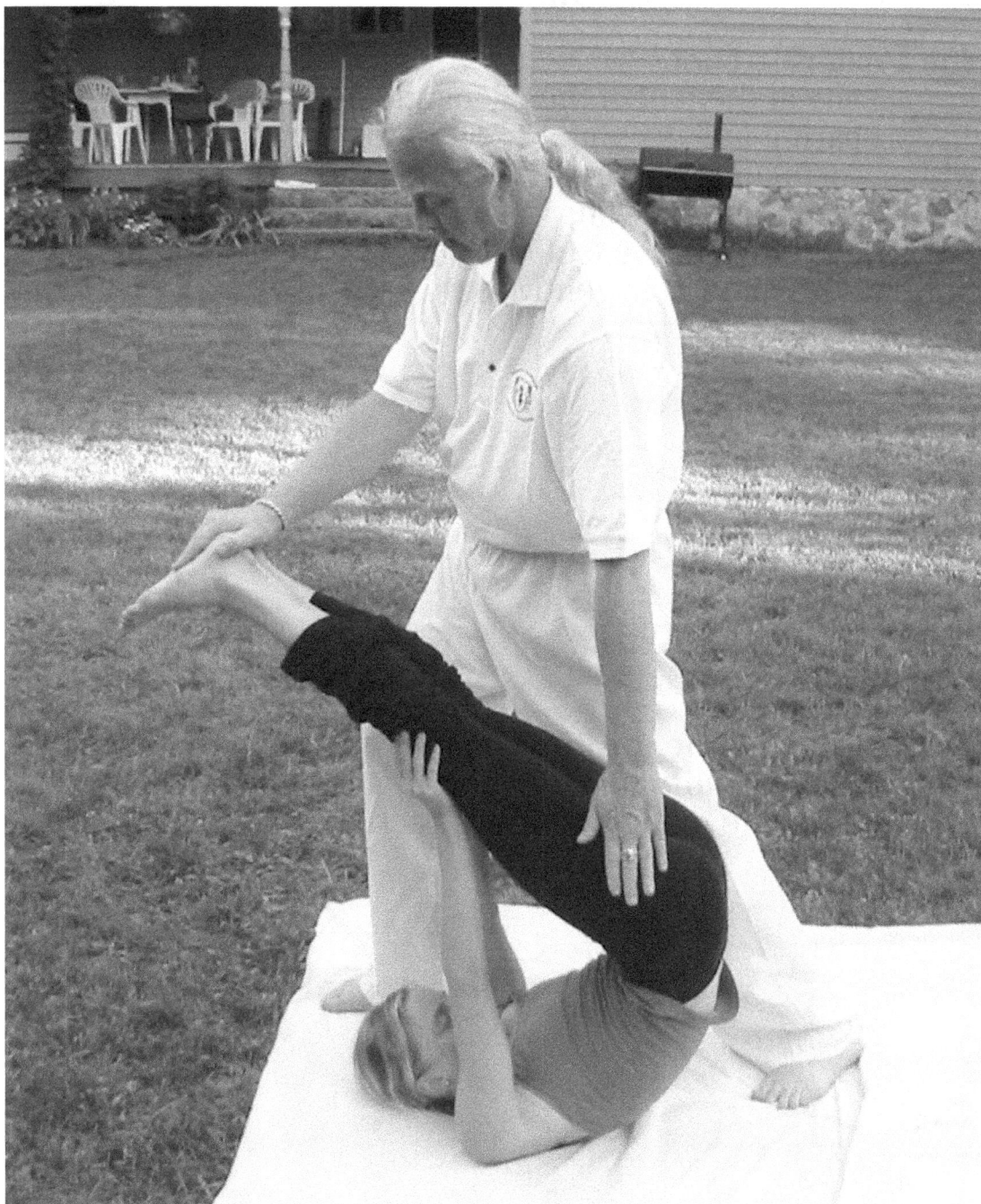

Proper execution and form in the Supported Shoulder Stand (Position #25, page 60) illustrates Center of Gravity and balanced easy posture. The Therapists is strong and centered where the client is most vulnerable.

Section One: Feet and Leg Lines

1. Supine Posterior Foot.

The therapist sits at the feet of the client and begins with Puja, preparing and grounding before touching. Begin with a warm-up of the feet and the legs. Palm Walk on both feet and work your way up both legs to the hip area and return to the feet. As you pass the knees both ways, palm circle gently to relax them.

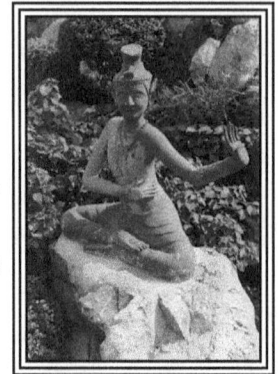

Fatao

The Feet and Leg Lines section is the Thai Foot Reflexology technique section. Thai Foot Reflexology can and is commonly used as a stand alone treatment or as an adjunct application to virtually any other type of healing expression or modality.

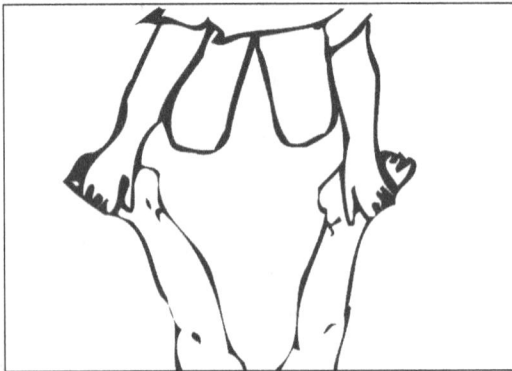

2. Begin the foot treatment with 6 points. (3 times)

Press each point and hold for 5 seconds each. Begin with #1 and move to #6 holding each one in turn.

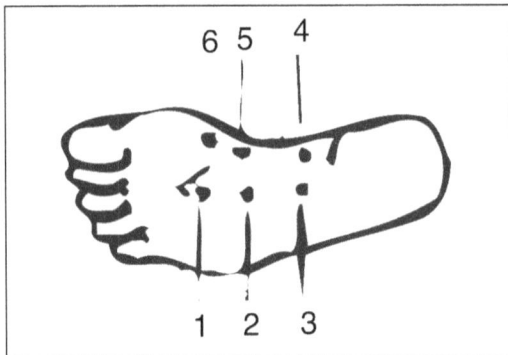

Point 1. In the middle part of the upper posterior foot. Same point as Kidney 1.
Point 2. Halfway from Point 1 to the heel.
Point 3. Just in front of the heel on the line with points 1 and 2.

Point 4. Medial of point #3 next to the heel on the
line from the big toe.
Point 5. Medial of point #2 also located on the big
toe line.
Point 6. Located at the proximal juncture of the
first metatarsal on the big toe line.
Repeat three times increasing pressure on the
first two circuits and slightly lighter on the last.
Finish with light palm pressing.

Note: The foot routine, steps #1-11 constitute a general reflexology treatment for the whole body. The Thai's have a long history of emphasizing the importance of feet points in treatments for every kind of disorder. For example see the feet of the reclining Buddha at Wat Pho, Bangkok.

3. Five lines
Begin at point #3, thumb press on the sole of the
foot on a straight line to each of the toes. Once
at the toes, lightly twist them doing thumb circles
to the tip then squeeze the ends before slipping
off the end. Finish with light palm pressing.

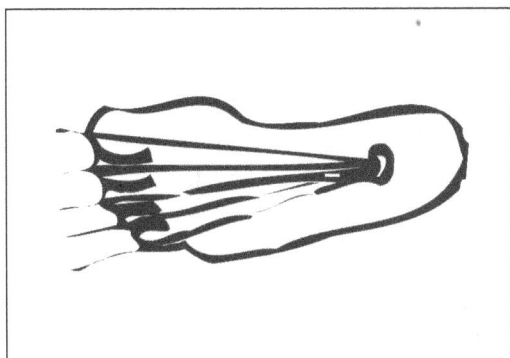

4. Supine Anterior Foot - 4 lines
Warm up the top of the feet with palm presses from
the ankle to the toes and return.

(Lang Tao)

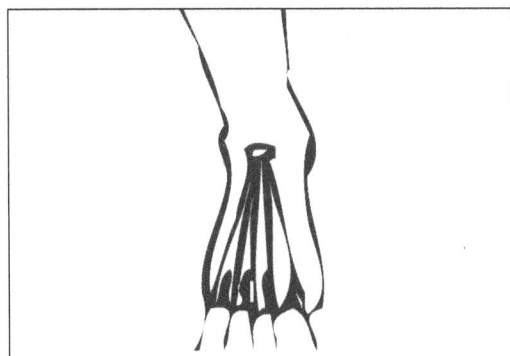

Apply thumb pressure at the medial juncture of the ankle and hold for 5 seconds.
Thumb circle between the toes four lines. Thumb circles on the toes, pinch them lightly and slide off. Finish with a series of palm presses again 1,2,3,2,1.

Note:It is not illustrated but the practitioner should thoroughly thumb press and palm press the feet between each individual step.

5. Supine Interior Arch - 5 points
Following the line of the arch work 5 points holding each for 3 seconds, perform this only once. Finish with palm pressing.

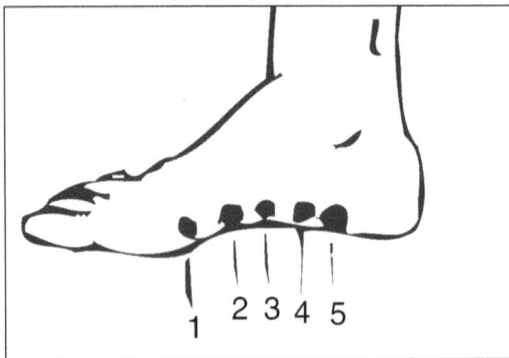

End bi-lateral foot section ... now work each foot, one foot at a time.

6. Supine Foot Rotation
Lift and support the foot with the hand, sliding your leg underneath for additional support. Place one hand under the heel and with the other, grasp the toes and rotate slowly 5 times in each direction.

(women left, men right)

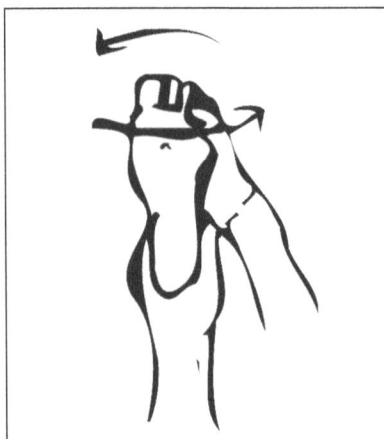

7. Supine Foot Stretch and Rotation
Grasp the foot firmly from the outside and pull while leaning back - this gently twists and tractions the foot. Pull in three positions beginning close to the ankle and moving distally toward the toes. Change hands and pull in three positions from the inside as well.

Note: Flexing and stretching the ankle, enhancing its rang of motion may positively impact a variety of disorders. Potential problems such as sprains and strains, calf pulls, shin splints and Achilles tendon injuries, foot stress, ankle and arch complaints are reduced.

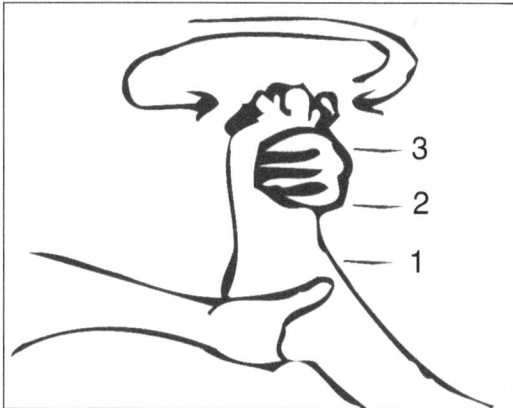

8. Finish by pulling the toes individually.
Before you actually pull the toes, gently circle them both ways to relax.
Change Feet and repeat Steps 6, 7 and 8 on the opposite foot.

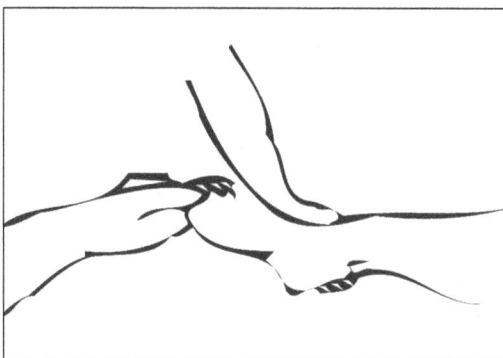

9. Supine Plantar Press

Palm press the feet in three positions then return 1, 2, 3, 2, 1.
The pressure is applied in such a way as to stress the feet in line toward the floor at ankle, arch and toe.

Note: Primarily affects the Tibialis anterior and extensor digitorem muscles.

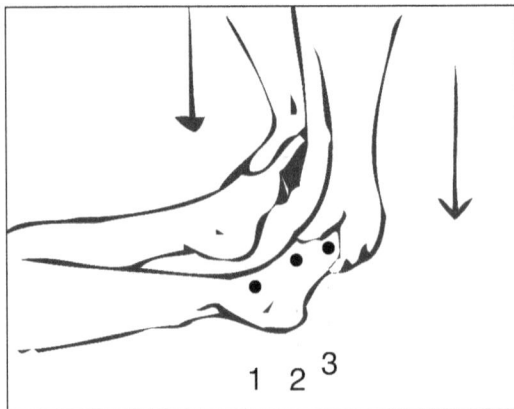

10. Supine Dorsi Press

Grasp the toes and press upward toward the shins in a series of three. Light, firm then light pressure.

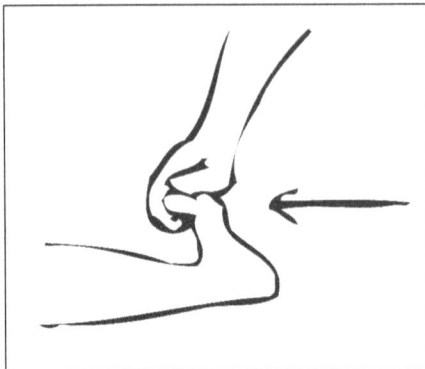

11. Cross the Feet and Press
Cross one foot over the other and use reinforced palm pressure to press the toes toward the mat. Repeat 3 times; light, firm, light.
Finish with Palm Walking pressure from the feet moving upward to the hips and returning once again to the feet. (Warm-up)

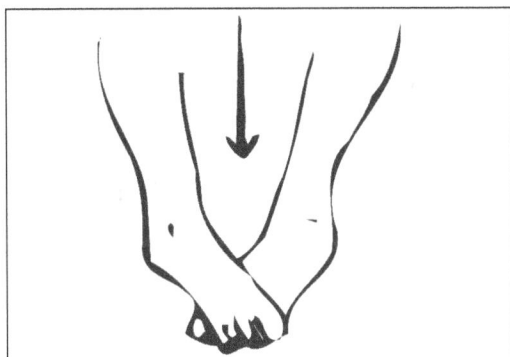

.... Begin Leg lines.

12. Supine Medial Leg (upper and lower)
Sit opposite the leg that you intend to work and reach across. Spread the legs slightly apart and warm up the medial leg.

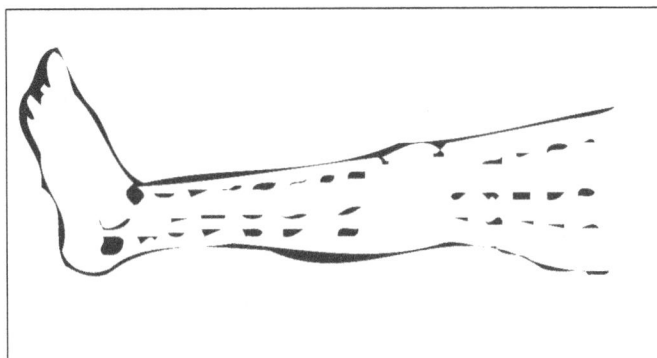

Leg Warmup:
PW IN
PW Out
PW In
Follow Down

Stretch the working leg. Then warm it up with alternating palm pressure. Begin with the hands at ankle and hip. Work inward to the knee then out again. Return inward to the knee and follow down to the ankle. Stretch the foot with both hands.
Line 1. Thumb walk from the ankle to the upper thigh. Return downward to the ankle.

Line 2. One thumb length medial to line #1. Thumb walk from the ankle (medial malleolus) upward to the femoral pulse then return to the ankle.
Line 3. One thumb length medial and posterior to line 2. Thumb walk from calcaneous or heel upward to just below pelvis and then return using the same method.
Finish by palm walking from groin area to ankle where you then stretch the foot.

13. Supine Lateral Leg (upper and lower)

Massage the leg closest to you. Warm up the lateral leg by stretching and palm walking as in treating the medial leg lines.

Leg Warmup:
PW IN
PW Out
PW In
Follow Down

One thumb lateral of Medial Line 1.
Line 1. Thumb walk from ankle to the hip and then return to the ankle.
One thumb length lateral to Line 1.
Line 2. Begin four fingers above (cranial) the lateral maleolus and thumb walk to hip and then return to the ankle.
Line 3. One thumb length lateral and posterior to line #2. Thumb walk from calcaneous to just below the gluteal area and return.

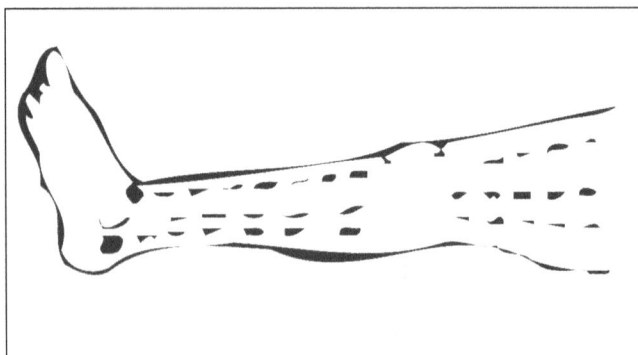

14. Open The Wind

(Bput Bpa tu lom)

Kneeling to the outside of the client's hip area, take the lower hand/palm and place it close to the inguinal area below the pelvic region, feeling for the femoral pulse. Once the pulse is located, place the upper hand on top and shift the body weight forward until the pulse diminishes. Hold for 10 as you shift backward, releasing the pressure slowly.

Finish by Palm Walking from the hip area to the foot.

Change side and repeat steps #12, #13, #14

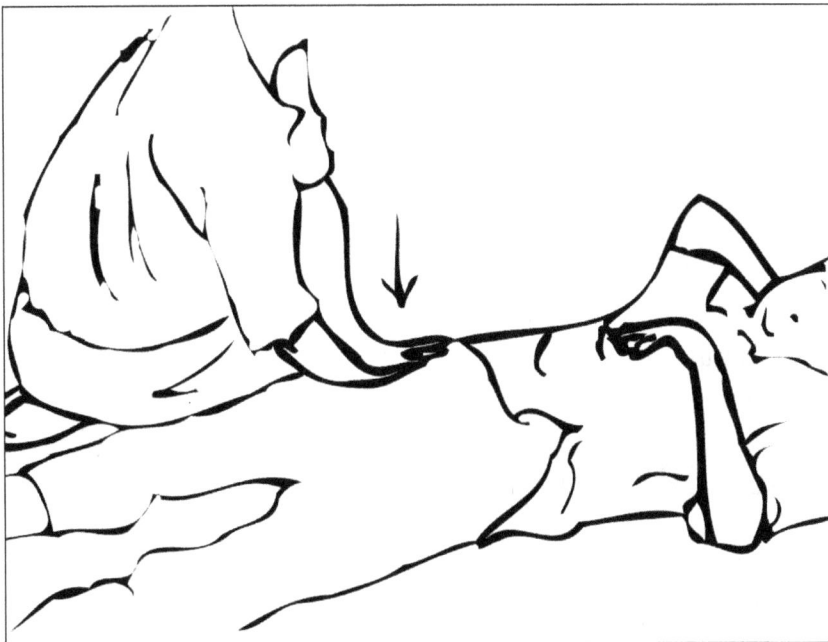

Synopsis: Feet and Leg Lines
Puja and Warm up

Step 1. Stretch feet

Step 2. 6 points (bottom, start with middle line)

Step 3. 5 lines (bottom, start with pt #3)

Step 4. 4 lines (anterior, top foot, start at ankle)

Step 5. 5 points in medial arch

Step 6. Rotate foot (one side at a time)

Step 7. Pull foot (3 Positions, both sides)

Step 8. Pull toes

Steps 6-8, do one foot at a time... Begin with left foot for woman and right foot for the man.

Change sides and repeat 6, 7 & 8.

Step 9. Press to floor

Step 10. Press to shin

Step 11. Cross and press

-- Change and repeat.

Step 12. Medial 3 lines (Running Thumbs on far leg)

Step 13. Lateral 3 lines (Running Thumbs on near leg)

Step 14. Open the wind

Change sides and repeat 12, 13 & 14

Repeat the Warm-Up (Step #1)

Remeber Northern Motto:
When in Doubt... Press it out!

Section Two: Supine Leg Stretching

15. Supine Medial Leg

(Technique: **Fa meung**)

The leg to be massaged is bent outward toward the side. Warm up both legs briefly from the feet to the inner thigh region with light palm walking pressure. Concentrate on the medial aspect of the bent leg with alternating palm pressure in three position

Stances are either a modified lunge as the Sen lines are on top of the body part being worked or kneeling and sitting on heels and knees.

1. Foot and thigh (Bottom of the foot and medial upper leg, 3 pts.)
2. Calf and thigh (3 pts on the calf and repeat same 3 points on the upper thigh)
3. Thigh and thigh (Palm heels tight together, same three points, fingers pointing in opposite directions in "**Butterfly** Palm Technique", 1, 2, 3, 2, 1

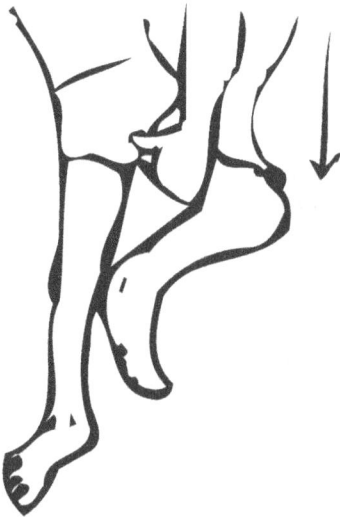

4. Repeat step #15.2 above (1, 2, 3, 2, 1)
5. Repeat step #15.1 above (1, 2, 3, 2, 1)

Finnish at the feet.

Ya Na Ka in Four Positions:

16. Supine Posterior Upper Leg
A. Push the leg outward to 90° and take the ankle with one hand. Raise the ankle of the bent leg and work the 3rd inside line of the posterior thigh with the heel of the therapist's outside foot.

(Technique: Dang ka - similar to Ya Na Ka of the Southern School)

Four Positions:
16. A. Single Leg Press
16. B. Lock 1 leg
16. C. Walking
16. D. Lock both legs and pull with hooking fingers.

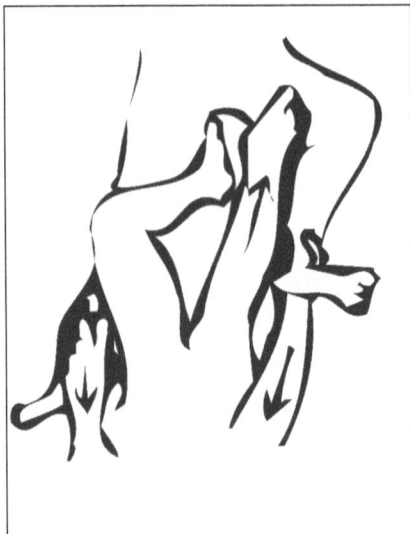

The resting leg (inside) of the therapist is relaxed and lying across the outstretched leg of the client. Massage posterior leg line with the outside foot three times beginning at the juncture of the knee and working to the groin area. Stay close but not touching the genitals. In general, you will find that most clients can take a good bit of pressure with this method. However, as always, be considerate of the comfort and tolerance of the client.

You may vary the actual application of pressure from light to strong by pulling with the hand in concert with the pushing motion of the feet.

Breathe and exhale as you push. Try to see even your foot press as an extension of your prana and breath.

B. Supine Posterior Upper Leg, Locked Position

Note: Affects the Adductor Magnus, Vastus Medialis, Biceps femoris, Semitendinosus, Semimembranosus

Begin in the same position as Technique #16. Grasp the bent leg and raise it up and over your outside leg. Turn the foot so that it will "Lock" against your leg. Now bring the inside leg to massage the posterior upper leg.

The proper technique is much like driving a car with a clutch.

While holding both heels firmly with both hands, alternate pressure between the foot. The outside foot is firmly placed behind the bent knee and the floating or free foot moves from there to the groin area and back. Work the line three times.

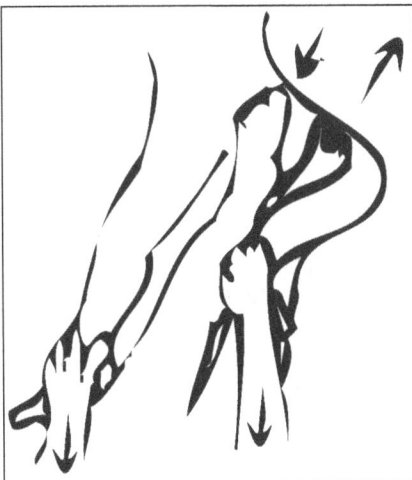

C. Supine Posterior Upper Leg, Walking Position.
Begin in the same position as in Technique #16. While holding both ankles, literally walk on the medial thigh with both feet. Work from behind the knee to a position near the groin three times.

Note: The reference technique by technique of performing a specific number of repetitions is for the basic routine only. The therapist may adjust the number of repetitions and their intensity completely according to the needs of the particular client.

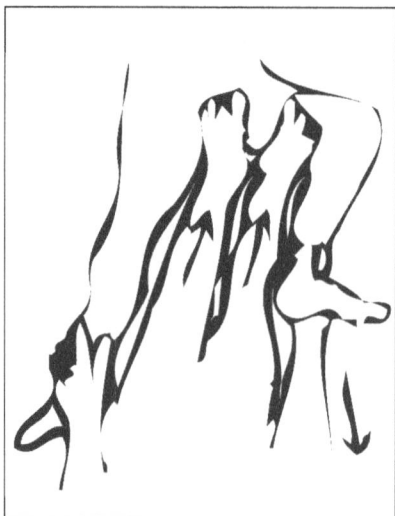

D. Supine Anterior/Posterior Upper Leg Combined
Begin in the same position as in #16. Bring the bent leg all the way up and over both of your feet which are placed on the posterior thigh. Scoot forward bending your legs until you can reach over to work the number one line of the lateral thigh. Use the "Hooking" technique and work the line from the hip to the knee.

NOTE The reference technique by technique of performing a specific number of repetitions is for the basic routine only. The therapist may adjust the number of repetitions and their intensity completely according to the needs of the particular client.

NOTE: Affects the Adductor Magus, Vastus Medialis, Biceps Femoris, Semitendinosus, Semimembranosus Rectus Femoris, Vastus Medialis.

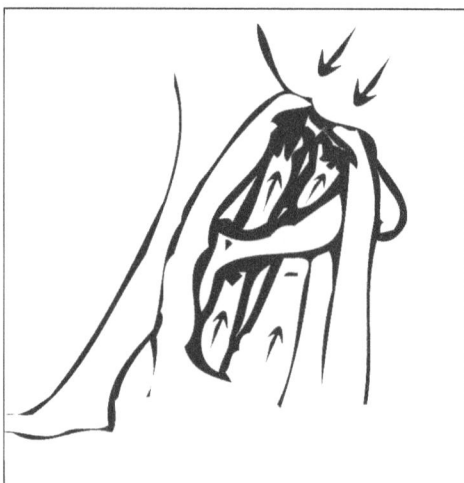

Now use the "Walking Hook" technique on the same line after this a further variation of treatment could be to use percussion techniques.

17. Supine Anterior Upper Leg (Sao Nong: Raised Bent Knee Position)

A. Lines #1. Raise up and bend the knee, sliding the heel toward the buttocks. Slide up close and capture the foot between your knees. On the lower leg, pull and give a stretch first. Then reach around to massage both the inside line #1 and the outside #1 lines with "walking Hook" technique. As you pull remember to work from your center and lean back to create pressure. Work from the hip area and move up the anterior leg, alternating pressure between hands.

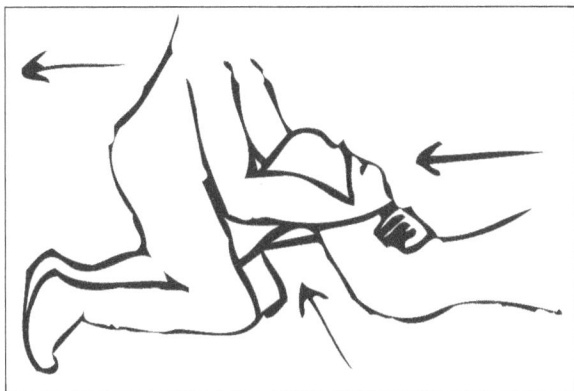

SAO NONG or Phoo Khao

NOTE: Affects Rectus Femoris and Tendinous attachments at the hip area and the knee.

Six Positions:
17. A. Line 1. Anterior Upper Leg with Walking Hook.
17. B. Lines 2. Upper Leg with locked fingers and Vise Palms.
17. C. Lines 3. Lateral and medial lines with crossed fingers and lever thumb.
17. D. Posterior leg line with Thumb Walking.
17. E. Posterior lower leg with Hooking Fingers.
17. F. Anterior & Lateral lower leg with locked palms pressing in and down.

B. Lines #2 Clasp the fingers together interlocking them. Lean forward far enough place the palms of the hands on the Anterior thigh. Press the elbows together to create pressure and work both inside #2 line and the outside #2 line from the hip area up to the sides of the knee. This creates a bilateral pressing or vice like effect with the palms.

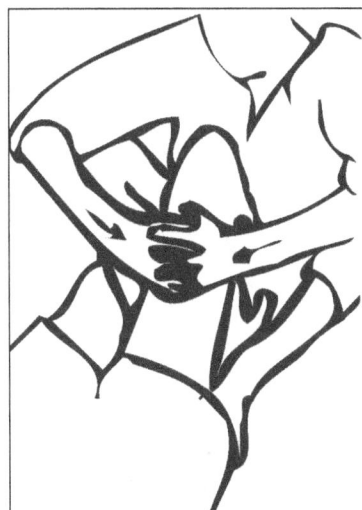

Sao Nong, Step #2
NOTE: Affects the Pectineus, Adductor longus, Sartorius, Rectus femoris, Vastus lateralis, Vastus medialis.

C. Lines #3
Clasp the fingers and turn the palms outward. When the thumbs are extended they should point downwards. Reach forward over the upright leg and working upward from the hip, massage the #3 Inside Line and the #3 Outside Line simultaneously. The thumbs create a bilateral pressing effect similar to that of the palms in #17B, but more specific.

Sao Nong, Step #3
NOTE: Affects the sartorius, Vastus Medialis, Gracilus Adductor Longus, Tensor facia latae, Ilio tibial band

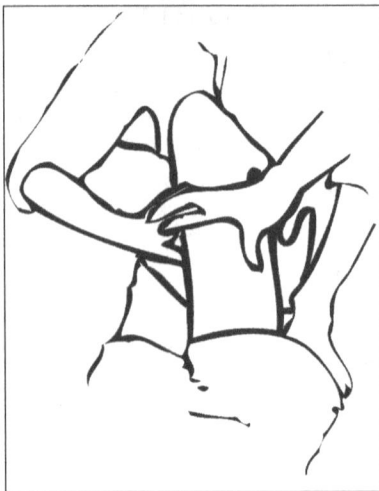

D. Posterior Lines, Upper Leg
In the Sao Nong Position, place the thumbs up close under the knee. Using Reinforced Thumb Technique work down the center of the posterior thigh one time. Next use Thumb Walking Technique up and down the line several times to relax. Use less pressure while thumb walking.

Sao Nong, Step #4
NOTE: Affects the Biceps Femoris, Semitendinosus, Semimembranosus, Adductor Magnus.

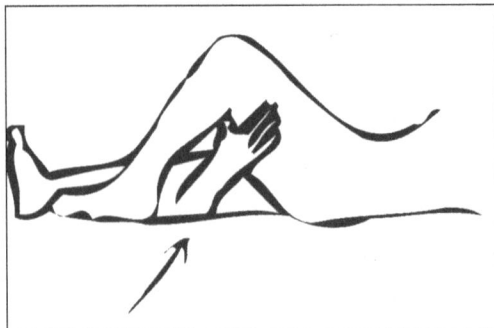

E. Posterior Lines, Lower Leg

With the knees locked firmly around the ankle, slide backward slightly. This pulls the client's foot forward creating enough space to place the fingers at the knee joint. Use Hooking technique with the fingers as you progress downward to the Achilles tendon. Pull from your center as you lean backward to create pressure.

Next, still using hooking technique, alternate pressure from side to side as you work down the line one time.

Sao Nong, Step #5
NOTE: Affects the Gastrocnemius, Achilles tendon, Soleus

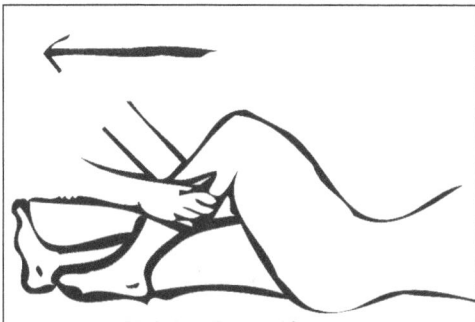

F. Anterior and Lateral, Lower Leg

Without changing sitting posture, clasp the finger is Vise Technique and pull the calf muscles (gastronemius). Pull three positions, top, middle and lower calf.

Sao Nong, Step #6
NOTE: Affects the Anterior Tibialus, Peroneus Longus.

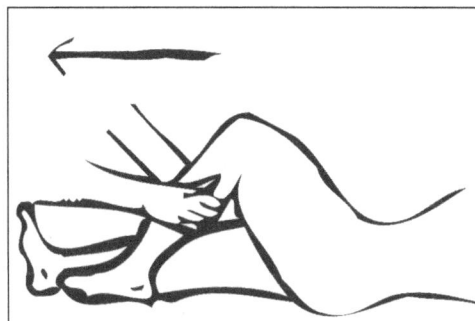

18. Dak Wukao (Vertical)

A. In the Lunge position step forward with the outside leg to crate a pocket. Place the client's foot in that pocket resting against the front of your hip. Support their leg with the raised knee and with a hand on their knee. As you slowly move your weight forward in a controlled lunge type of motion, use the inside hand to work 3 points on the medial thigh of the outstretched leg. Work each point three times in concert with the stretching.
Point 1. Femoral point. Point 2. Mid thigh. Point 3. Knee. Hold Lom (pt #1) for 15 seconds then release slowly.

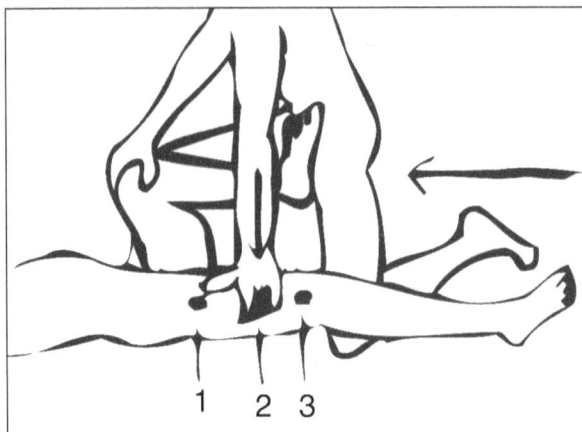

(Lunge Position)
Dak Wukao
Three Steps:
18. A. 3 Pts. Extended Leg

18. B. 3 Pts. Bent Leg (Posterior upper, leg line)

18. C. 3 Pts. Medial Leg (With the bent leg adducted)

Step #1, Lunge & Press 3 Pts Lower Leg.

CAUTION: Always work within the reasonable tolerance of the client. Do not ever force the body.

NOTE: Affects the internal hip muscles and rotators, Pyramidalis, gracillis, Adductor Longus, Pectineus and Sartorius.

B. Use both palms to work the sides of the posterior upper thigh while stretching the leg. Massage 3 points. 1. Lower thigh near knee, 2. Mid thigh, 3. Upper thigh.

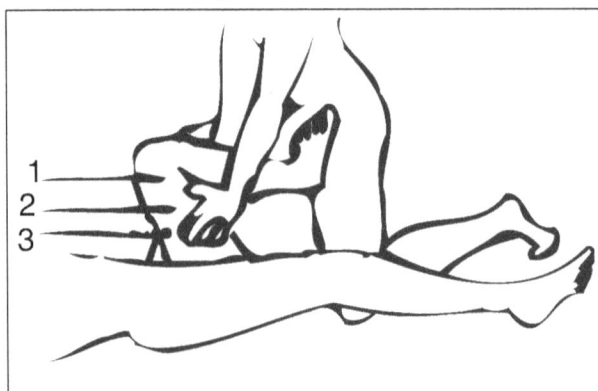

Step #2, Lunge & Press 3 Pts. Posterior upper leg.

C. Turn the knee out as close to 90° as the flexibility of the individual will comfortably permit. Work 3 points on the inner thigh three times. Point 1. Lower thigh near the knee, Point 2, Mid thigh. Point 3. Upper thigh

(Horizontal)

Step #3, Lunge & Press 3 Pts. Medial leg.

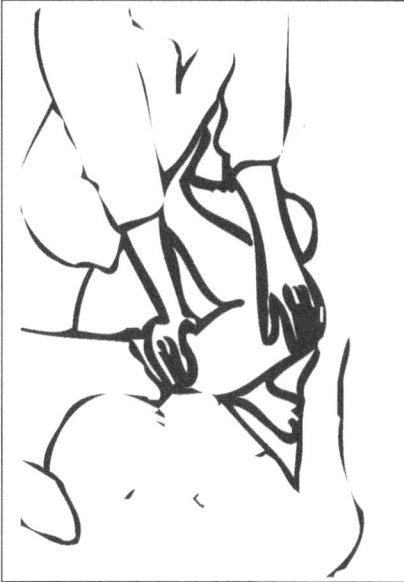

Recover the leg back to the center line before pushing the heel up and forward into step #19, Straight Leg Stretch in the lunge position.

19. Straight Leg Stretch (In Lunge Position)   (vertical position)
While kneeling between the feet lift the leg by
grasping the ankle with your inside hand. Once the
leg is in a vertical position work the posterior upper
leg lines with palm and thumb pressure with the
outside hand.

You may finish with a percussion technique on the
#3 outside line by changing hands and striking with
your inside band.

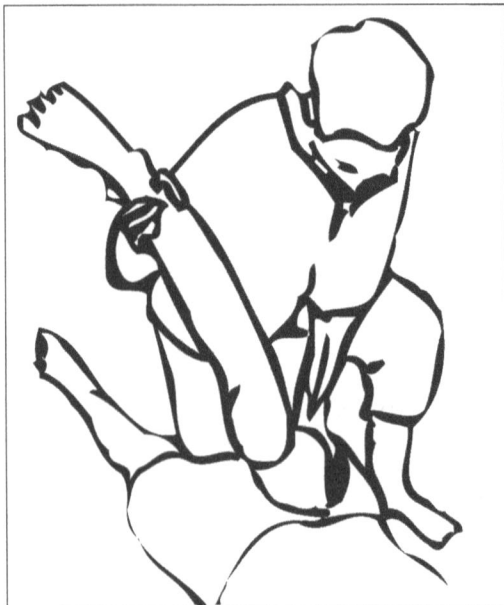

Work three
positions with palm
pressure while resting
the leg toward the
sternum. Point 1.
Lower thigh; Point 2.
Mid thigh; Point 3;
Upper thigh.

20. Vertical Dang Ka (YaNaKa)

Vertical Dang Ka is a variation on the ya na ka technique. You raise the bend leg to 90° and work the posterior upper leg lines with the feet, while at the same time pulling with the hands on the ankle. The two major variations of this technique are
A) Working the lines with one foot while the second presses at the hip.
B) Working the lines with both feet simultaneously.
   Massage 3 points, two times. Point 1. Lower thigh right in knee joint;Point 2. Mid thigh, Point 3. Upper thigh, close to the hip.

Rock back on your bottom to get into this position from the Straight Leg Stretch.

Basically this is the same technique as Ya Na Ka but with the knee pointing directly up wards. Pressure is still on the posterior leg Sen lines, Bladder Meridian and Hamstring muscles.

Added benefits include: tractic and decompression of both the knee and the ankle joint. Additionally this big pressure also moves a lot of fluid and is helpful with Edema and or swelling, fluid retention in the legs ad lower extremity.

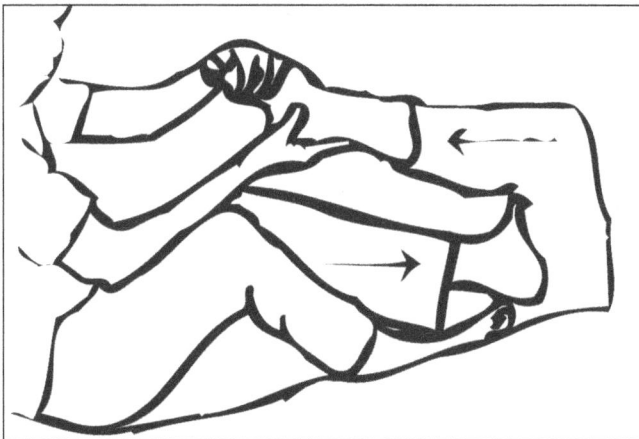

21. Traction the hip and leg

The setup is similar to that of Vertical Dang Ka. The bent leg is raised upright to approximately 90°. You press your inside foot directly on the base of the leg at the floor. This has your foot covering the glut/hip/upper leg. The outside leg is bent and held close for support.

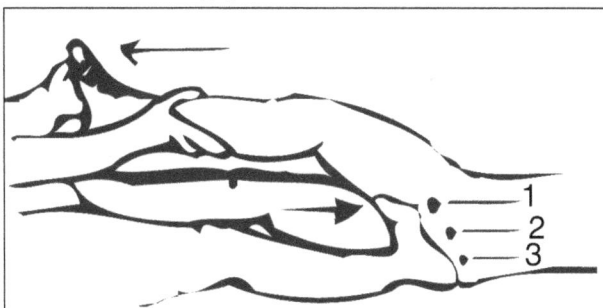

POINT 1. Pull the ankle and leg with your hands as you simply lean away from the client. The ball of your foot provides the pressure at the hip. When properly executed your weight provides the traction more than the pulling action of the arms. Keep breathing.

POINT 2. Raise up and push the leg forward, slightly ahead of the original starting position. As you do this keep your foot in place and stationary. Repeat the leaning and pulling movement.

POINT 3. Repeat same procedures as before; however, push the leg farther still to cause the ball of your foot to fall on Point 3.

3 Posteerior Hip Points...

The Ball of the foot, behind the toes, is the primary contact point for applying or directing the pressur. Keep your toes back and do not let your foot collapse as it can cause a strain injury to your ankle or foot if not properly set up.

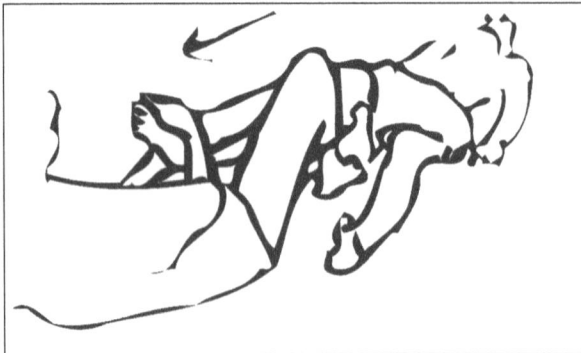

22. Supine Anterior Lateral Upper Leg

Massage the first and the second line on the lateral thigh with Fa Meung technique. Bend the knee inward and the foot to the outside in a "Hurdlers Stretch" type of position. A flexible person's knee may go to the mat; however, if unable to get the knee down, kneel closely and support the bent leg on the top of your thighs.

Begin by bracing the lower palm on the client's knee and palm pressing with your upper hand. Work from the hip to the knee in increments of about one hand width. Repeat pressing three times before using hitting or percussion on the upper and lower leg in the same position. Finish with a gentle stretch of the knee toward the mat. Watch the client's face and their breathing for signs of any strain. In which case, this is your cue to release the stretch slowly.

After releasing to a relaxed position, gently rock the leg and palm circle the knee joint ten times in each direction to relax the fascia and the connective tissue of the knee joint before proceeding to the next procedure.

(**Dak Kha**-inward knee position)

NOTE: Affects tensor fascia latae, illiotibial band, Vastus lateralis, peroneus longus, tibialis anterior, rectus femoris and psoas major.

Dak Kha, Four Steps:
1) **Test** (For range of motion)
2) **Palm** (Bi-lateral Palm Press the Sen)
3) **Hit** (2 Hand Hacking and percussion on Sen)
4) **Stretch** (Explore release)

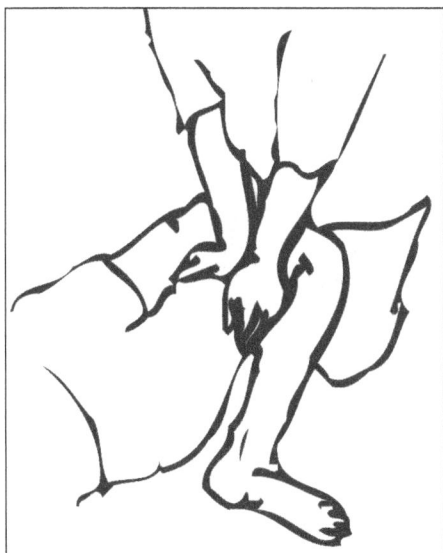

23. Straight Leg Stretch (Lateral Position)

In a kneeling position use your outside leg to push or press the client's leg outward away from the body. Move the leg gradually being sensitive to any felt resistance. Once the leg is extended in the stretched position, simply plant your foot firmly to hold the leg securely in the proper position.

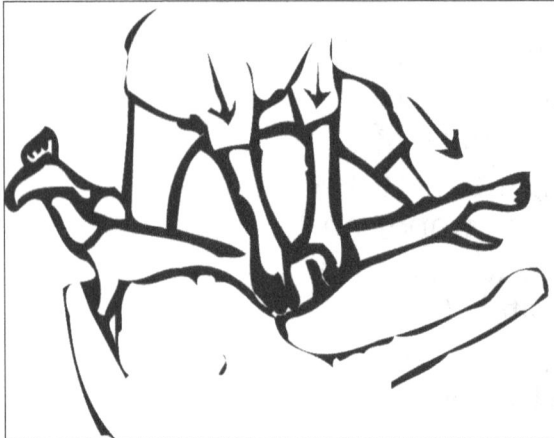

1) Palm Press 3 points on the upper thigh beginning one hand width above the knee. Hold each point 10 seconds or longer.
2) Hold the femoral or wind point for 30 seconds.
3) Palm walking lightly over the medial thigh. Recover the leg inward by dragging your foot inward to you.
4) Thumb Walk Sen 1 and 2 (medial) 3 times

Swing out! keeping the clients leg on top of your foot. Inch your foot forwardforward until the inner leg comes into tension.

(Horizontal position)

NOTE: Affects the biceps femoris, gracillus Achilles tendon, soleus, gastroe remius, and generally stretches the hamstringL

Lateral Straight Leg Stretch, 4 Steps:
1) PP 3 Pts.
2) PP Lom, 30 count
3) PW Medial leg lines
4) TW Sen 1 & 2 (medial)

24. Supported Straight Leg

Rest the ankle of the straight leg on the top of your raised thigh. Take the ball of the foot in the lower hand and massage the anterior upper leg from the hip area to just above the knee. Press and hold 3 points on the anterior thigh each for 5 to 10 seconds.

Finish with a series of leg checking. Bend the knee slightly and then pull the heel outward with a snap. Not too hard! Use just enough force to gently check or lock the knee into a maximum extension for a moment. There would normally be little or no pain associated with this technique.

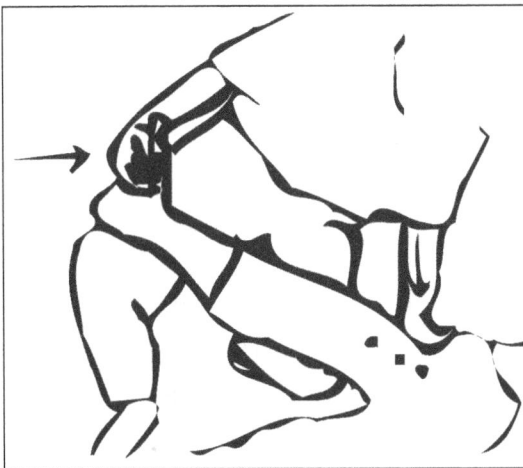

Change sides and repeat #15 (#15= Fa Meung on the opposite leg) Through #24 on the opposite leg.

25. Supported Shoulder Stand

With both legs raised and held together by the therapist, the client is instructed to relax and allow the therapist to press both feet together toward the head. The feet are returned to the vertical position and the client is instructed to lock the knees and to secure them in this position with both hands, their arms are also locked into place. Hold the ankles and press again over the client's head until the weight of the body is full onto his shoulders. Hold in this position for five seconds, then slowly release. Repeat the first step again with the client in a relaxed position. With a flexible client you may push the feet all the way to the face.

However, sensitivity to any discomfort or pain of the client is important. The therapist should walk forward, going with the stretch to avoid leaning and straining.

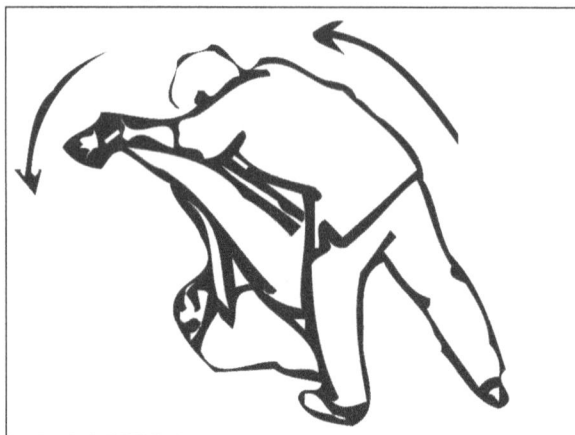

(Sarvangasana)

NOTE: This is a general stretch affecting the entire back and posterior hip musculature including the posterior cervicals and the hamstrings.

The supported shoulder stand is one of the three traditional postures thought to be able to stimulate Sen Sumana and perfect health for the whole body.

3 Easy steps:
1) Pull to your mid-section.
2) Turn and look
3) Push into position...

Remember... In any balancing position or inversion, you want to be able to be strongest and in the best possible position when your partner is at their most vulnerable and risky. Avoid positioning yourself so that you are strong at the beginning when the partner is safe and weak in the end where the partner is at risk.

Make sure your partner is breathing and there should be no pressure on their neck at all.

26. Supine Posterior Upper Leg and Crossed Leg Stretch Combined.

At the completion of the Supine Inferior Foot (standing position),

Leave the leg crossed and raise the upright leg and lean or set it firmly on the top of your outside shoulder. Reach around the upright leg to secure or grasp the foot of the bent leg. Press the posterior thigh of the bent leg towards the chest using palm pressure in three positions:

1. Upper thigh
2. Middle thigh
3. Lower thigh, just below the knee. Hold each point for 5 seconds each.

Lever against the resistance of your front leg.

Steps #26, 27 and #28 are performed the same as in Level Two (Southern Method).

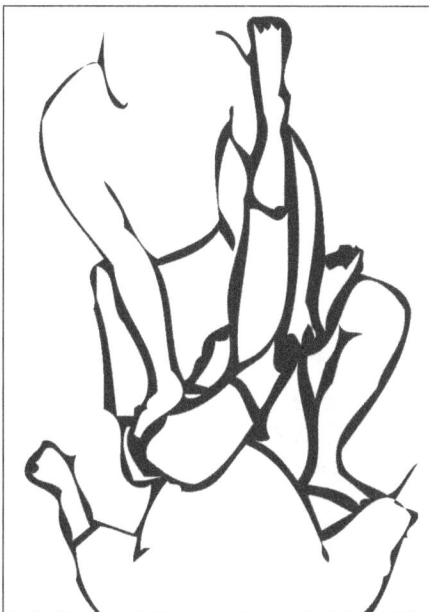

27. Supine Vertical Crossed Leg Stretch

(While standing)

With both legs upright in a vertical position, bend one leg inward crossing it over the upright leg at the knee. Step over the bent knee in such a way as to allow you to simultaneously secure that knee in place and to push the upright leg forward with the hands.

Go slow and repeat this movement three times.

NOTE: Stretching the muscles of the hip joint expands the possibilities for a free range of movement in the hip, pelvic girdle and the lower back; the flexibility of the hips even affects the knees and upper cervical areas. This posture affects the hamstrings, internal rotators of the hip and the lower back musculature.

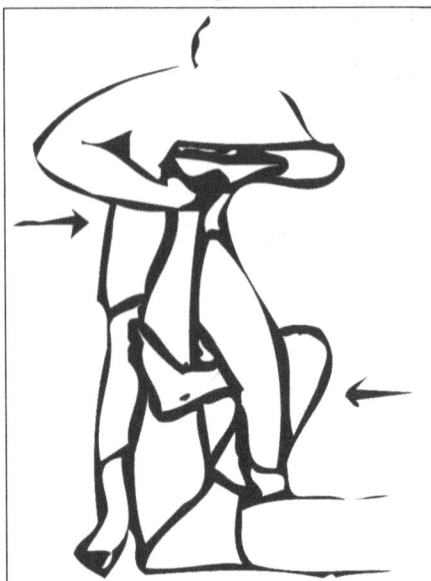

28. Supine Inferior Foot

Place the client in the Supine Vertical Crossed Leg Position and move your body behind the vertical or upright leg to support the leg against your hip. Once securely in position relax the inferior foot with forearm rolling technique from heel to toe. Next press kidney one (K1) point on the foot with the elbow for 5 seconds. Massage the 6 points on the inferior foot with the elbow and then roll the foot out again with the forearm. Finish with light hitting or percussion of the foot and posterior thigh.

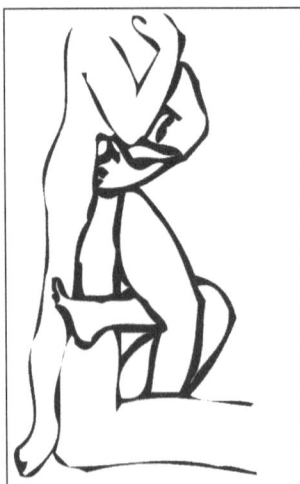

Change sides and repeat #26 through #28.

29. Knee Press to Posterior Thigh
Begin with the legs extended upright in a vertical attitude. Stand close and buckle the knees of the client inward toward their chest while holding onto the ankles.

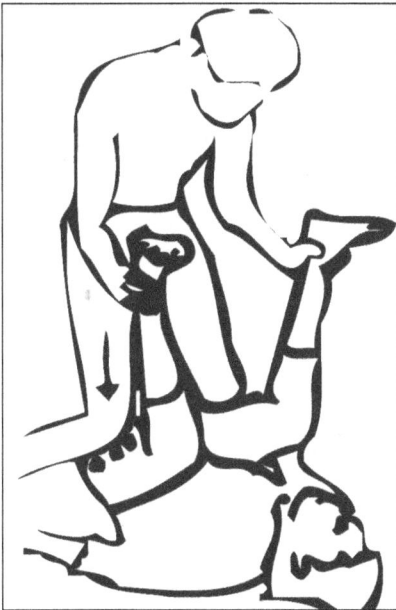

Rock on! Start low, extend your arms and rock your weight forward onto the knees to control the extension. Exhale as you more forward bringing energy attention, consciousness, breath and pressure onto the Sen lines on the back of the legs. Have the client exhale at the same time.

NOTE: This posture is contraindicated for menstruation, pregnancy, heart disease.

Kneel forward directly onto the posterior upper leg. Massage three positions, upper, middle and lower with knee pressure. Work each point 2 times.
A more advanced technique is to rock forward completely supporting your body weight on your knees pressing the client's thighs right down to their chest.

As your moving into the pressure position try to keep your arms straight and use your bodies mass to create the pressure. Exhale as you rock forward.

30. Supine Straddle and Press

Begin with the legs extended upright in a vertical attitude. Stand close and spread the legs wide enough to allow you to step over them placing your feet beside the torso, close to the armpits. Bring both of the client's legs around in front of you, bending them as you do so. Place the soles of their feet together and gently press the feet in three positions.

A. Press the feet toward a point located over the head.

B. Walk backward toward the hips and then press the feet toward the face.

C. Remain standing in the same place and press the feet again toward a point over the head. Press at each position gently 3 times while bending your knees as well - work with the breath and sink as you exhale, rise up and release as you inhale.

If the client has difficulty getting into this position. Don't force it. Remeber to keep the overall pressure within the reasonable tolerance of the client. In this facilitated reverse Butterfly posture it is the posture that does the work and provides the benefit.

All of the Asana or postures we facilitate are therapeutic in and of themselves. It's never just about range of motion!

In every Asana the 5 attributes or causative factors we seek are:
1) Energy
2) Intention
3) Consciousness
4) Breath
5) Pressure

Pressure, the last listed, is just the little finger on the proverbial therapeutic hand.

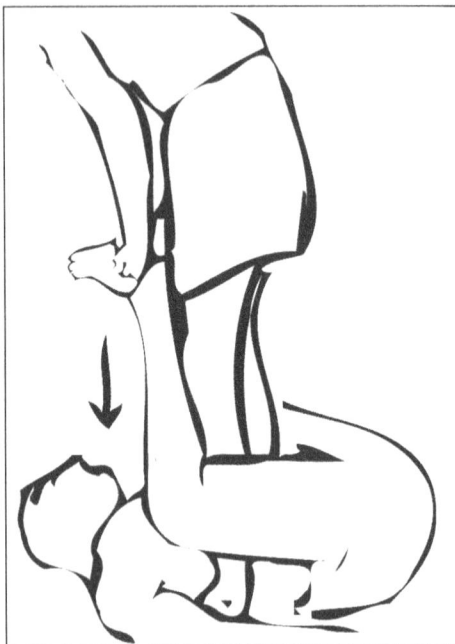

31. Straight Leg Pull Up

Begin with the client's legs extended upright in a vertical attitude. Stand close and grasp both of the client's arms at the wrists. Use a combination of a leaning and a pulling movement to pull the client upright into the forward bending position. Repeat, three times.

(Ubhaya Padangusthasana)

Protect your back by useing proper bodymechanics when performing any kind of lifting. Bend your knees, push your hips forward, keep your torso upright and lift with your legs.

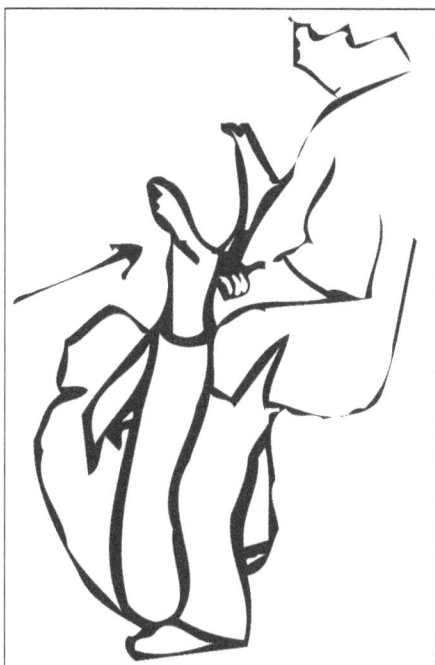

32. Crossed Leg Pull Up

Begin with the client's legs extended upright in a vertical attitude. Stand close. Bend and cross both of the client's legs and support them against the front of yours. Grasp both of the client's arms at the wrist and use a combination of a leaning and a pulling movement. Pull the client upright into the forward bending position. Repeat three times.

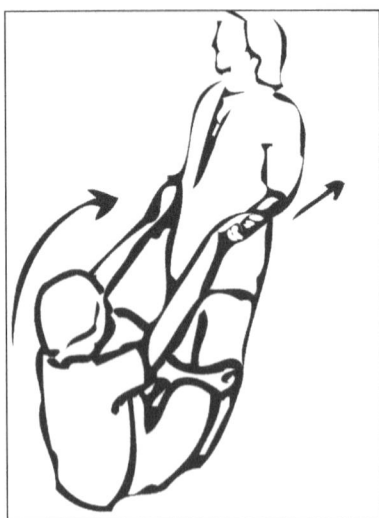

33. Seated Shoulder Press

Pull the client upright into the S.P. or Seated Position and walk around to their rear. Standing right next to them - your legs are close enough to support their back. Lean forward and press 4 points equally along the top of the shoulder with bilateral thumb pressure. Work these points with two different hand positions.

Seated Shoulder Press Five Positions:

A) Palm Press, Fingers to back
B) Palm Press, Fingers to front
C) relax the back
D) Hitting the back
E) Brush Out

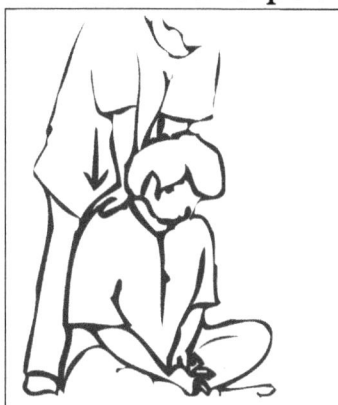

A. With the fingers of the hands on the back side of the body

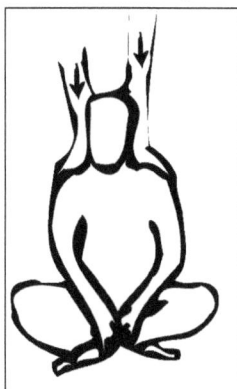

B. With the fingers of the hands toward the chest or front of the body. Work each point 2 times.

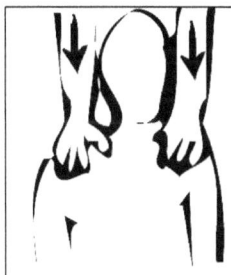

C.Relax by palm pressing from the neck out to the shoulder then returning to the neck. Then palm walking down the sides of the spine to the low back area and then returning again to the neck.

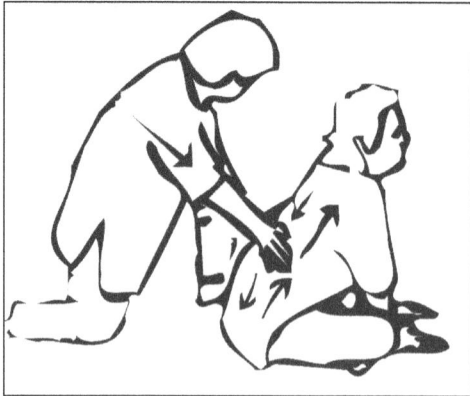

D.Finish by hitting gently across both shoulders lightly. Some light palm circles are nice.

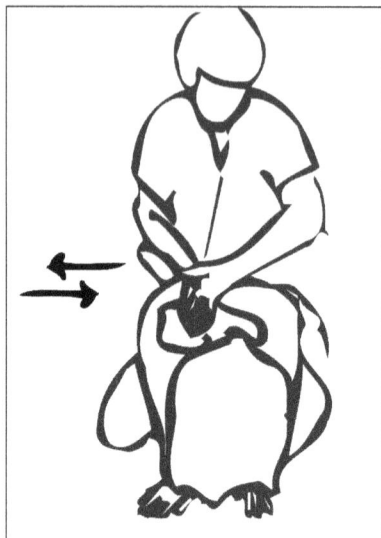

E. Lastly, use Finger Tip Brushing Technique outward from the spine several times.

Synopsis: Supine Leg Stretching

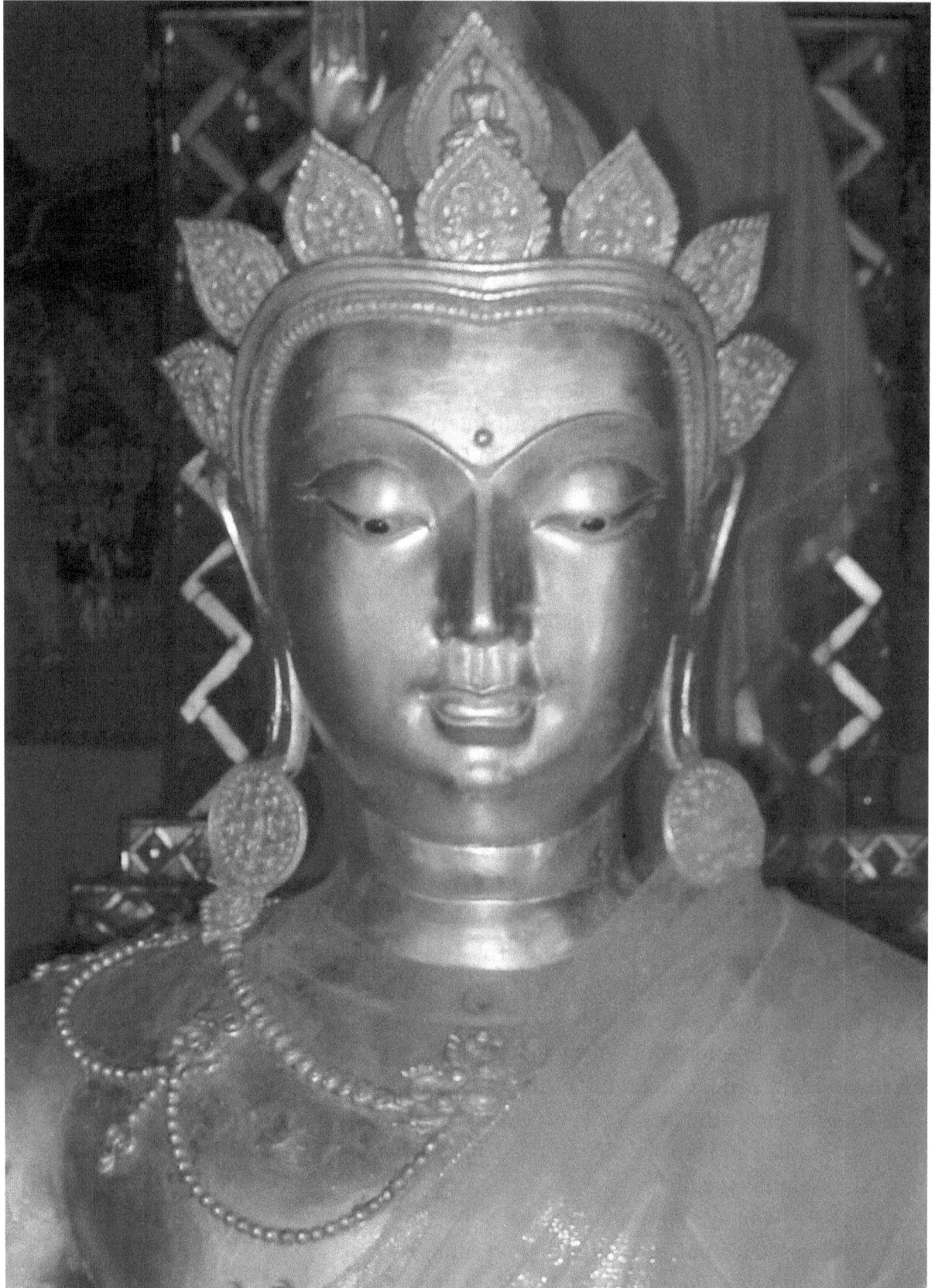

Ancient Buddha's of Wat Hariphunchai, protect and bless healing traditions.

Section Three: Abdominal Technique

The Thai believe that the stomach is the center of the body's universe and, as such, is the "window to health."

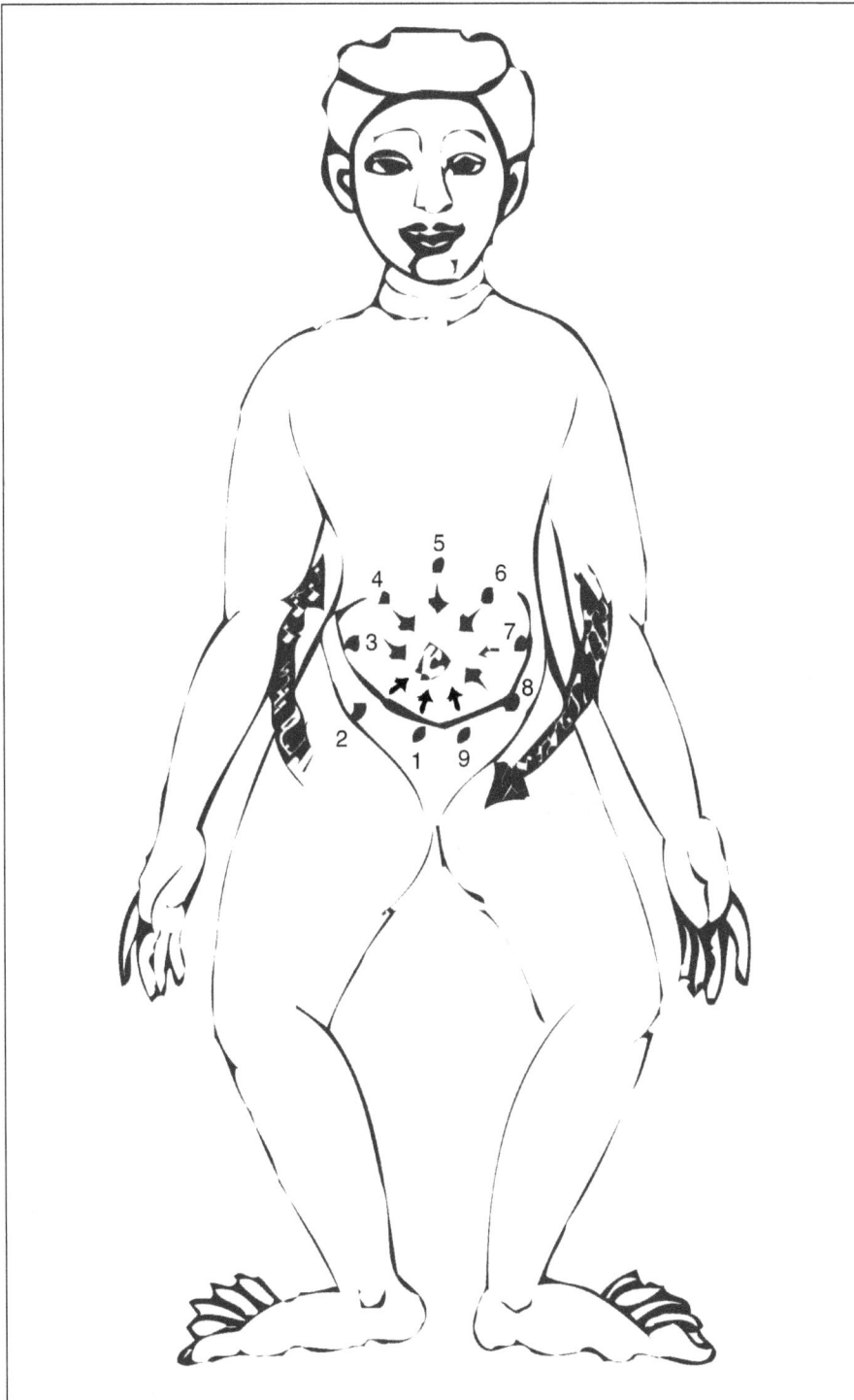

Step 34. Nine Points

Sit on the right side for a man and on the left side for a woman.

Hold your hand over sadung or the abdomen and focus energy and light there. Relax and breath slowly. Before you touch this sometimes quite sensitive area—pay respect and honor the spirit.

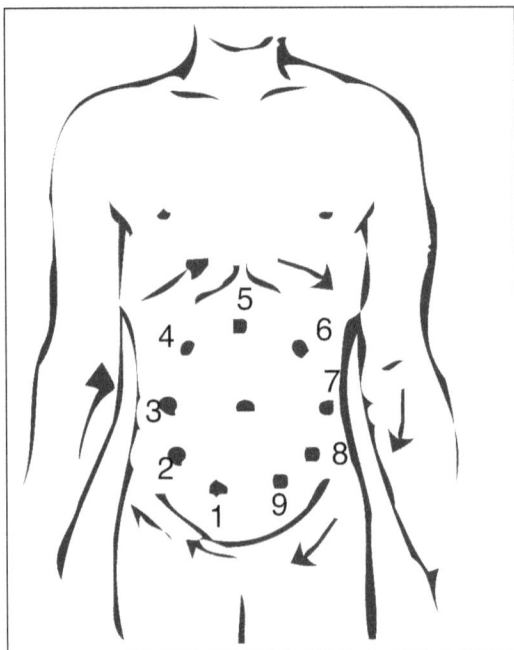

A. Make small light palm circles beginning at the navel, then moving clockwise from point number one. Circle around the periphery of the abdominal area finishing at point number nine.

B. The second part of nine points treatment is to use push and pull technique on each point.

Beginning with the palm heel of the hand on point number one, push the palm slowly down and inward, moving the pressure toward the navel. As you come to the navel, release the pressure and rock the hands over onto the finger tips. Press inward on the opposite side with the finger tips that are held rigid. Drag or pull them back toward the point being treated. Gradually release the pressure and move on the next point.

Move slowly while focusing on the breath. Press inward as the breath is released and lift the hand away as the client inhales. As you move around to each of the nine points feel free to move and adjust your own body position. Some therapists will rotate around their client like the hands moving on the face of a clock.

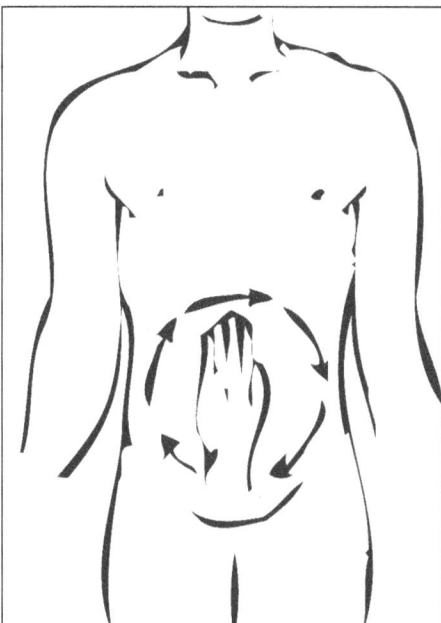

C. Finish or complete the application of pressure to nine points by pressing over the navel area with a cupped hand. Now relax further with some gentle circles with the palm. Nine points begins and ends at the center.

35. Six Points

Straddling or having one leg over the client's abdomen work the six points in pairs bilaterally. Points 1 and 2 are one thumb length above the navel and one thumb length lateral to the center line. Points 3 and 4 are lateral to the umbilicus and points 5 and 6 are one thumb length below points 3 and 4.

Keeping in line with the general guidelines of following the breath down - work each point two times.

Finish with relaxing palm circles of abdomen.

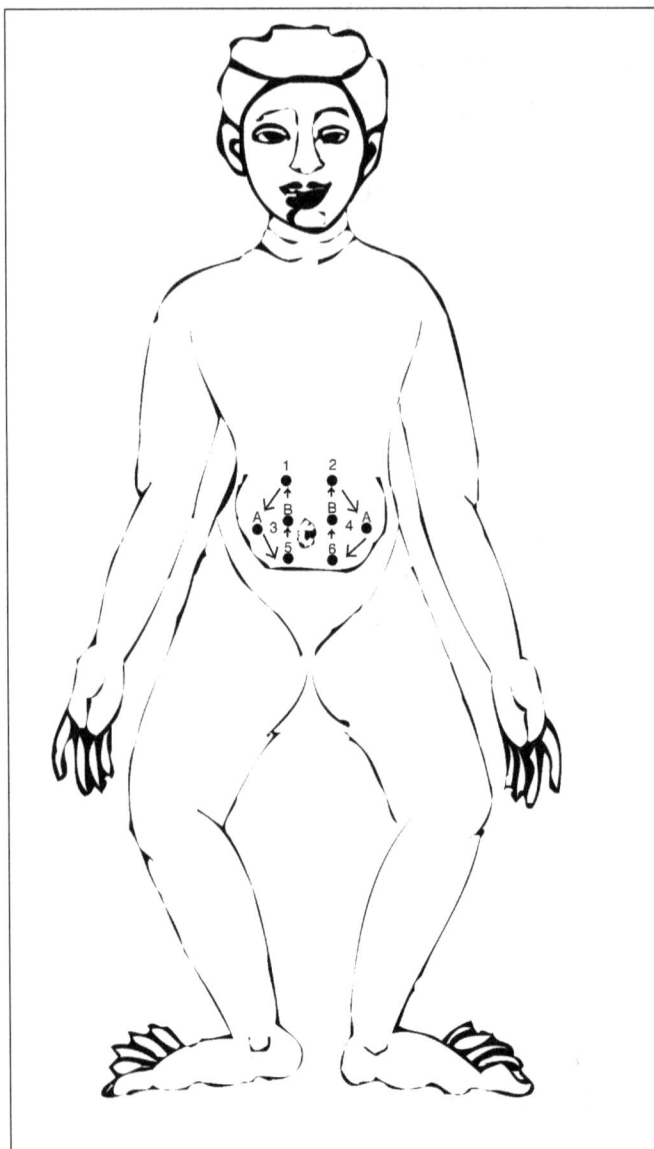

Section four: Anterior Torso/Arm

36. Anterior
Begin low on the sternum with finger circles from the sternum to clavicle three times. Again with finger circles begin at the manubrium or upper sternum and massage outward under the length of the collarbone three times.

Continue working in this fashion the intercostal spaces between the ribs. However only work outward on the rib spaces.

Generally work above or just below the soft tissue of the breast.

Massage the lateral torso with palm circles from armpit to waist, down and up, three times. Use a loose big circular motion moving a lot of skin.

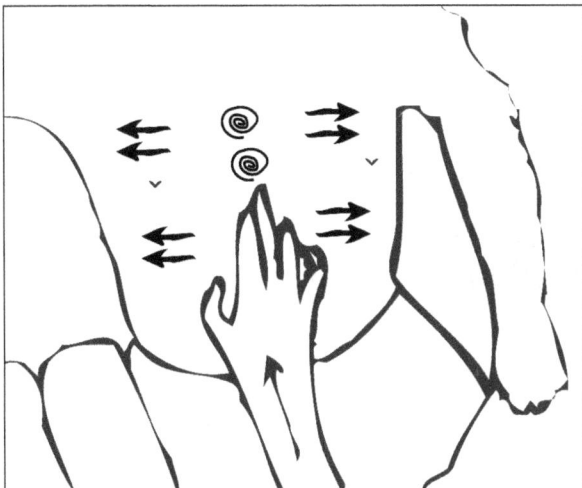

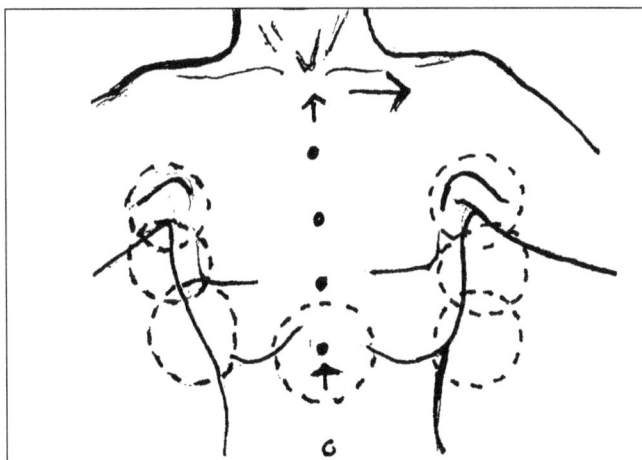

This technique also stimulates the movement of lymphatic fluid by addressing the lymph nodes of the upper torso and intercoastal region.

Finger Circles:
Up, Down, Up

Out, Back In, Out

This is the best area to include the Basic Breast Massage Protocal. Can also be done as a separate break out session. See breast Massage course or textbook for more information.

37. Anterior Low Back Stretch

While straddling the client's body reach around and under in order to work bilateral points along the spine with the finger tips. Lift and rock backward with your arms locked and straight. Work from your dan tien and lower back rather than pulling with the arms.

Finish by making palm circles on the lateral torso from the hips to the arms three times.

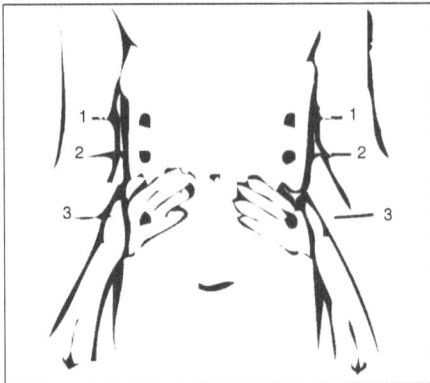

38. Shoulder Press and Pull

Palm press the two shoulder points #1 and #2 then #1 again before pulling with the Hooking Technique the three posterior points along the top edge of the trapezius muscle.

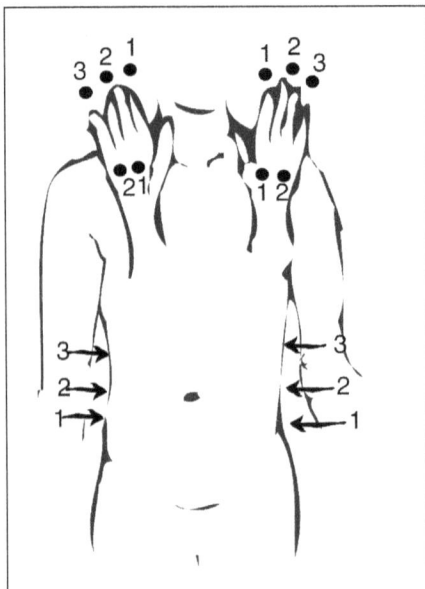

39. Anterior Medial Arm

First warm up the outstretched arm with gentle palm pressure and stretching. Use the same basic procedure as when working the legs. Walk in from shoulder and wrist to the elbow and then back out. Repeat one time then Palm Walk with both hands out to the wrist.

Thumb Walk out to the wrist from the axila with the client's wrist in the supine position. Palm Walk returning to the axila where you then hold the brachial artery point. Hold or press the point with palm pressure 10 to 20 seconds then release slowly.

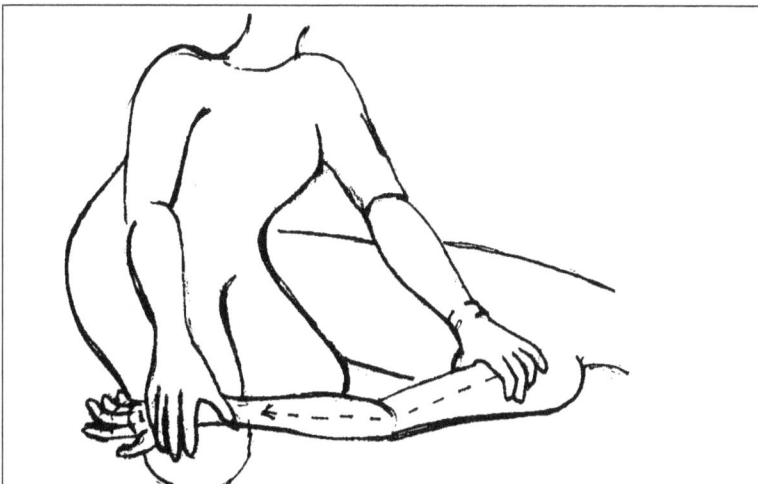

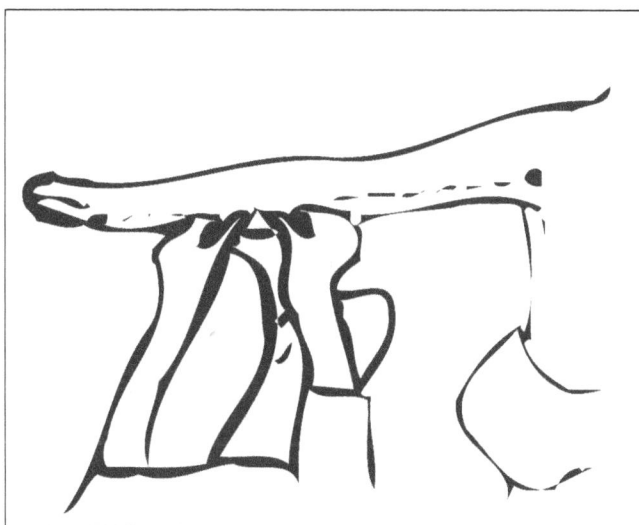

40. Anterior Lateral Arm

Note:(Supraspinatus, Infraspinatus and Teres Major)

First warm up the arm which is lying alongside the client's body with palm pressure and stretching. Use the same procedure as before. Walk the palms inward to the elbow, out to the shoulder and wrist and then return again to the elbow. Palm Walk both hands down to the wrist. Return to the crest of the shoulder and pressing on the medial deltoid locate the S.I.T. tendons. Thumb Walk from this point on the lateral shoulder to the wrist one time and then Palm Press the arm from the wrist upward to the shoulder.

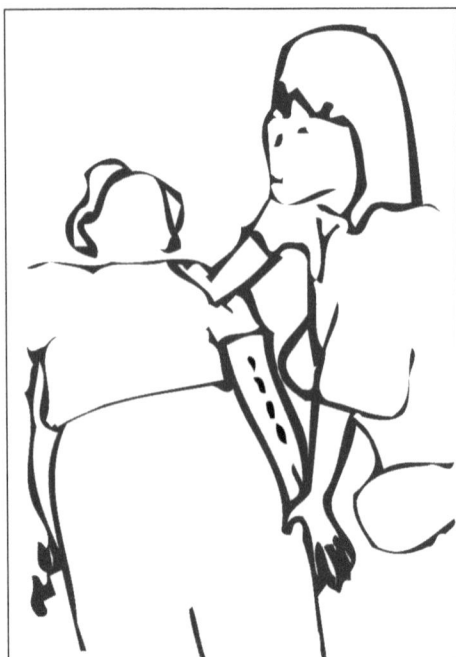

Section Five: Reflexology of the Hand

41. Supine Posterior Hand Six Points
Grasp the clients hand firmly and secure it by sliding the last two fingers of each of your hands between their fingers.

Begin by warming up with a general squeezing and pressing of their whole hand. Alternate pressing with both thumbs.

Once this is done hold each of the six points with a bilateral thumb pressure. First working the top two points, followed by the middle two and finally the bottom or most distal points. Massage each point three times. Please note how the hand treatments parallel the foot treatment.

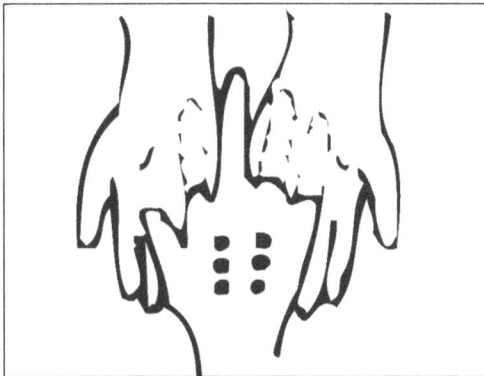

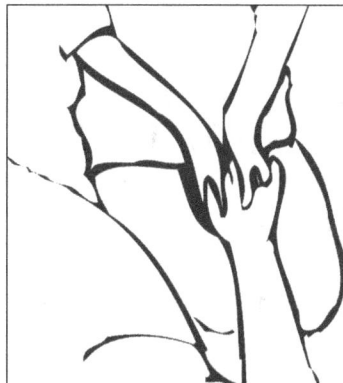

42. Supine Posterior Hand—Five lines.
Massaging from the wrist chakra point, use thumb circles to work the lines distally to the finger tips.

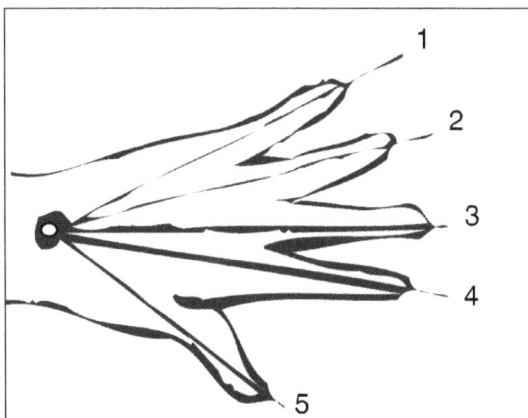

Chapter Five: Supine Position

80

Once on the fingers themselves use a pinching and rolling method pressing the finger between your thumb and first finger. Go back to the wrist point every time and continue until all five lines are done. Use the thumbs to randomly press or dance again all over the palm surface to complete "5 lines."

43. Supine Anterior Hand—Four lines

Turn the hand over (Pronate) and grasp the hand firmly in both of yours. Pull and squeeze generally with both hands. Begin at the top of the wrist at the wrist chakra or point, located between the Radial and Ulnar bones of the arm - where they meet the wrist itself.

Massage and press each of the four lines in turn, holding the terminal point between each finger or in the web of the hand, briefly. The lines run fairly between each of the metacarpals of the hand from the center point to the wrist.

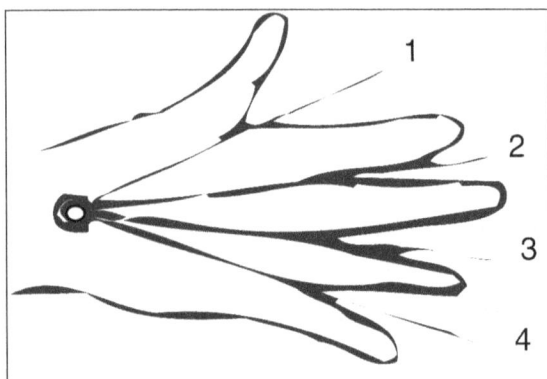

44. Passage Range of Motion on the Wrist
A. Raise the client's hand and slide the fingers of one of your hands between theirs while supporting the arm with your free hand.

   With an easy relaxed kind of motion rotate their wrist five times in each direction.

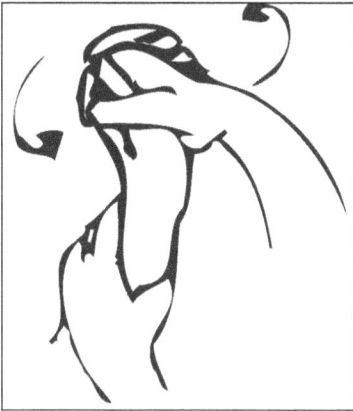

B. While the fingers are interlocked pull the hand toward you three times stretching the fingers.

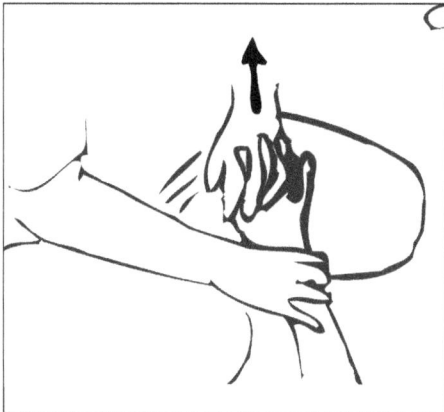

45. Pulling the Finger

Grasping each finger in turn between your first two fingers, relax by circling and then pull firmly along the longitudinal axis of the finger. This gives the fingers gentle traction. The joints of the fingers may make a popping or cracking sound, but this is not the intention of the technique. It is incidental to the technique. If the joint mobilizes or releases with an audible sound, fine, it it does not, that is fine also.

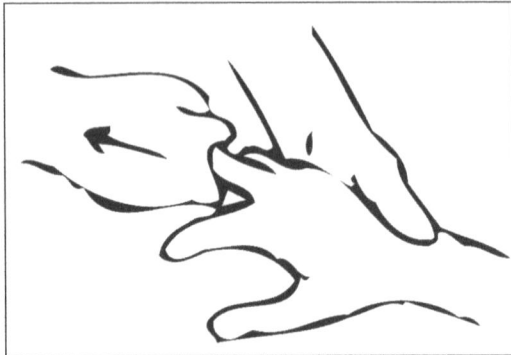

46. Stretch the Fingers

Fold the hand back and holding it firmly, rub and stretch the entire palm surface between your thumbs. Use the thumbs in opposition to create friction. It does not matter from which side you begin from; however, be sure to thoroughly cover the entire palm surface. This insures that you may stimulate and provide good coverage of the many reflex points in the hand which may affect the whole body as well.

Beginning with the little finger, press out and stretch each finger from the base of the finger outward to the tip.

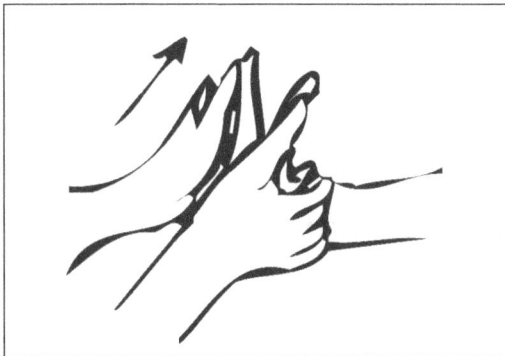

47. Supine Posterior Upper Arm

Raise the arm and fold it over placing the hand in an inverted position beside the head. Position your body in such a way as to allow you to simultaneously stretch the elbow and the anterior superior hip. Use a sinking motion directing the movement with the breath.

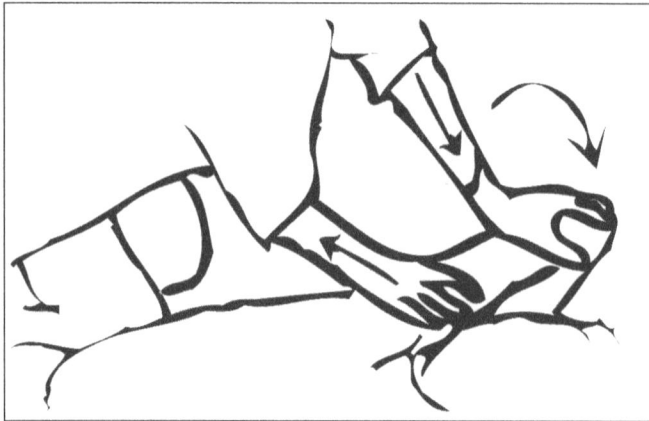

Retain the upper hand on the elbow and work the three anterior thigh points. Hold the first point or the femoral point for 5 seconds then release slowly.

Use the Tiger Hand Technique to squeeze and press alternately the posterior upper arm. Brace the elbow with one hand while pulling with the other. Work three positions from distal to proximal 1, 2, 3, 2, 1. Raise the arm, grasp the hand and give the whole arm a good shake. Drop the hand alongside the body.

Change sides and repeat steps #39 through #47

Do the other arm P. 76 to P. 84.

Section Six: Neck, Head and Face Routine

48. Supine Neck, Head and Face
A. Sit at the client's head and support the client onto the front of your legs. This places the back of the client's head in your lap. They are well supported in what generally turns out to be a comfortable and nurturing position.

Palm press outward on the top of the shoulders. Work the top of the shoulders from the neck outward with thumb pressure several times.

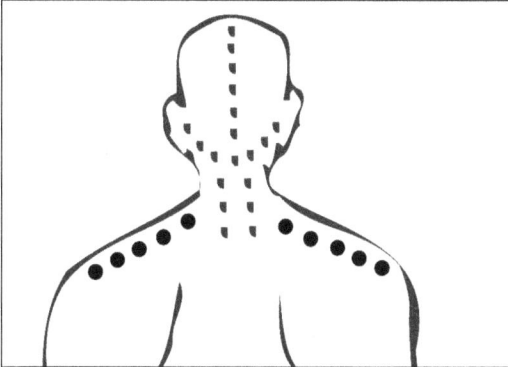

Reach under the neck and use a hooking technique working points alongside the next from the base of the occiput to the C-7 area. Work around the cranial base points of the occiput with finger tip pressure and then bring the finger tips together at the back of the head and work the center line from occiput to the crown several times.

B. With reinforced thumb pressure, work center line points from the crown point (Sahasara chakra) to the hairline. Walk the thumbs back to the crown and repeat this procedure three times.

Scrub the whole head lightly with all of the fingers and finish with gentle brushing and stroking of the hair.

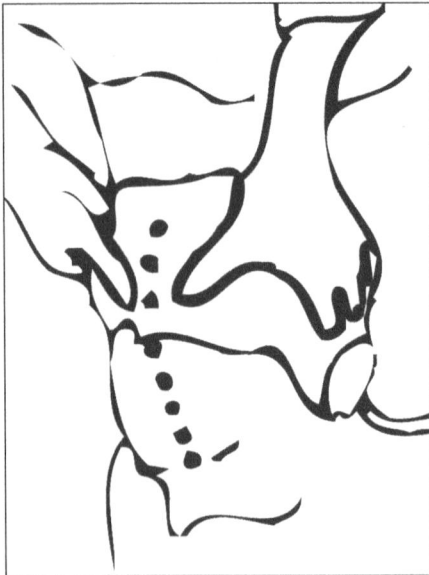

C. Facial Treatment.
Move to a seated or kneeling position in front of the client.

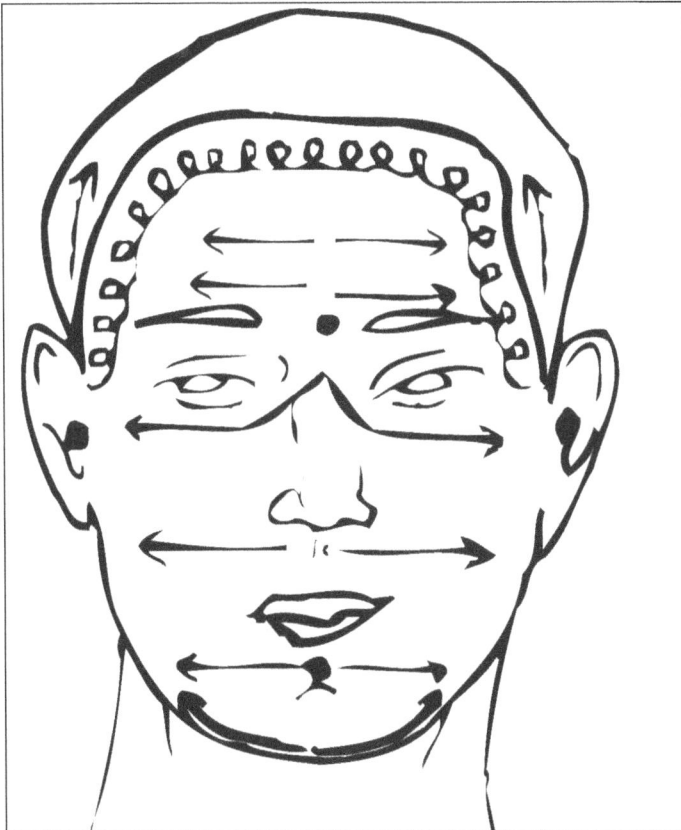

1. Massage around the hairline, using thumb pressure, three times.
2. With the thumbs, press out each line one time:
A. Mid-forehead
B. Eyebrow
C. Under eyes
D. Maxilla
E. Mid-chin
3. Press the ears closed and hold for five seconds, release quickly.

Relax the feet and the legs with palm walking from the ankles up to the hips, returning to the ankles and feet.

Step 32 x 3 Crossed Leg Pull up
Step 33 x 1 Seated Shoulder Press

Synopsis: Abdominal

Torso

Step #36: Up, down, up... out, back, out... down, up, down.

Step #37: Figer Circles up, down, up

Arm

Reflexology Hand

Arm

Change sides and repeat #39 through #47   Arm and Hand Section

Relax and finish with:

49. S.L.P. Medial Inferior Leg

1) The inferior leg and superior are warmed up with light palm walking pressure. Begin at the feet and work upward toward the hip. Now concentrate only on the inferior leg. Use the same technique or method as used before in the Supine Medial Leg (Step 15), palm press inward toward the knee then outward, then in again and outward to the ankle, stretching the foot.

2) Begin at the ankle thumb walking inside line #1 on the lower leg. Line #1 is directly medial, centered right on top of the leg in this position.

3) Thumb Walk line #2 on the lower leg, three times. Line #2 is one thumb length posterior of #1 at the top of the leg closest to the hip and one finger posterior at the ankle. Go up, down, up.

4) Now work the inside line #3 on the bottom leg three times.

The third line you work in the S.L.P. inferior leg moves basically upward along the most posterior aspect of the leg from the ankle to the gluteal area.

5) Hold the femoral or Lom (Wind Gate) at the top of line #1 of the upper leg for 20 seconds with reinforced palm. Release the point slowly.

Finish with both palms following each other down to the ankle and then stretch the foot again.

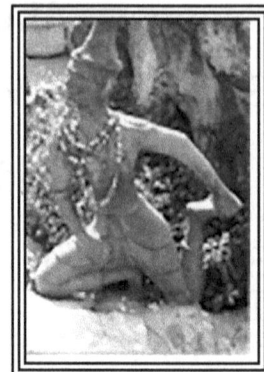

First Warm-up the medial leg

Note: Affects the Illiopsoas, gracilius, Sartorious, pectinus, Uastis medialis, gastrocnemius and soleus.

Medial Inferior leg, 5 Steps...
1) Warm-up the leg
2) TW Line #1, 3X
3) TW line #2, 3X
4) TW line #3, 3X
5) Hold Lom 20 count

Follow Down...

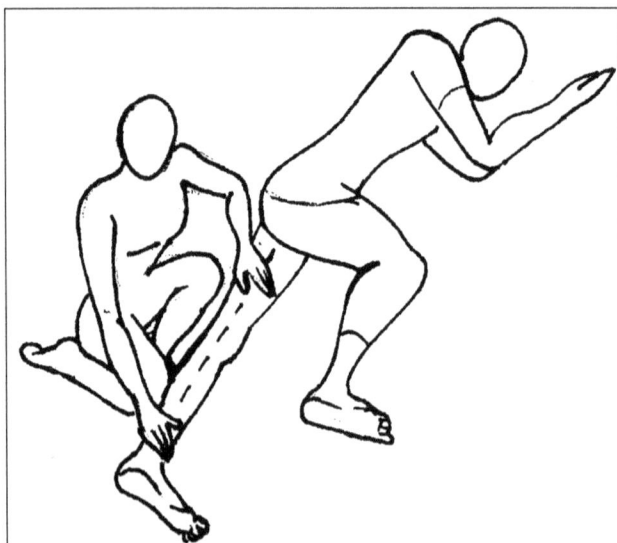

50. S.L.P. Lateral Superior Leg.

1) Warm up the leg properly with stretching and correct palm method. The palms move in, then out, in again, then follow down to the ankle.

2) Thumb walk the line #1 of the superior leg, 3X.

3) Thumb walk the line #2, 3X. This line is one thumb length posterior to #1, beginning in the depression just posterior of the greater trochanter.

4) Thumb walk the line #3, 3X. Line #3 is the most posterior line, directly down the back of the leg, from sit bone to heel.

Finish with the Standard Palm Pressing/Walking Technique and stretch the ankle.

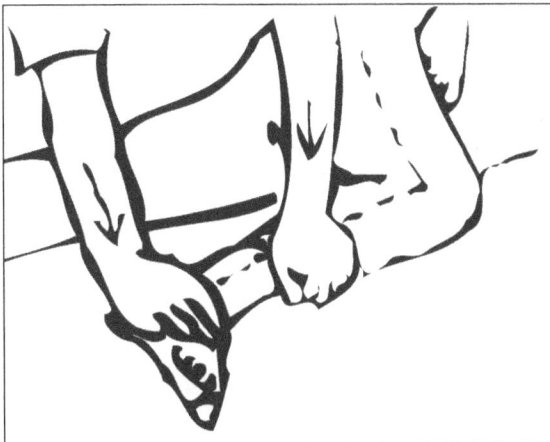

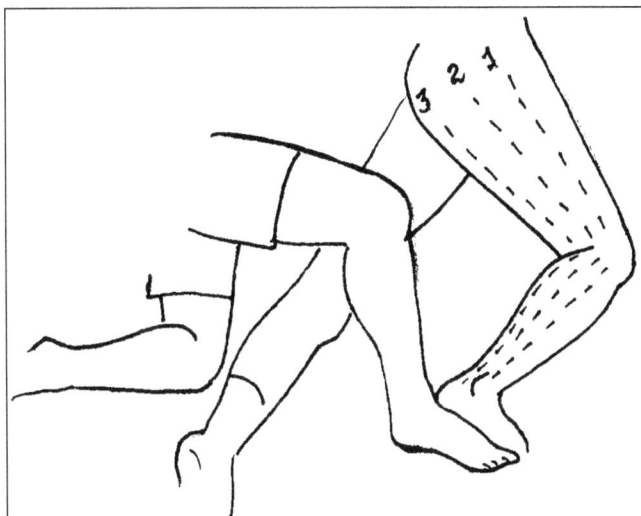

Affects the tensor fasciae latae, iliotibial band, vastus lateralis, lower attachment of gluteus maximus, tibialis anterior, peroneus longus, extensor digitorem longus, and gastrocnemius, biceps femoris muscles.

Lateral Superior Leg, 4 Steps:
1) Warm-up
2) TW line #1, 3X
3) TW line #2, 3X
4) TW line #3, 3X

Follow Down...

51. S.L.P. Superior Leg—
A. While sitting behind and below the client, Foot Press the superior posterior leg with your outside foot while supporting the ankle of that leg with a firm grip. Massage the posterior aspect in sections from behind the knee to the posterior hip.

(Ya Na Ka)

Note: Steps #51 A–D are the side lying variation of steps #16 A–D and essentially the same muscles are involved.

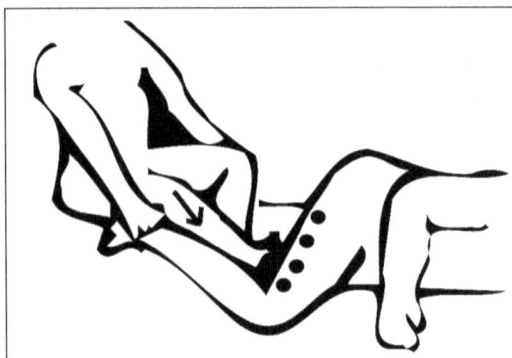

B. Lock the Leg over your outside shin and then Foot Press the posterior line again with your inside foot. Alternate pressure between the feet with a push and pull motion while tractioning the heel of the lockd leg with the outside hand.

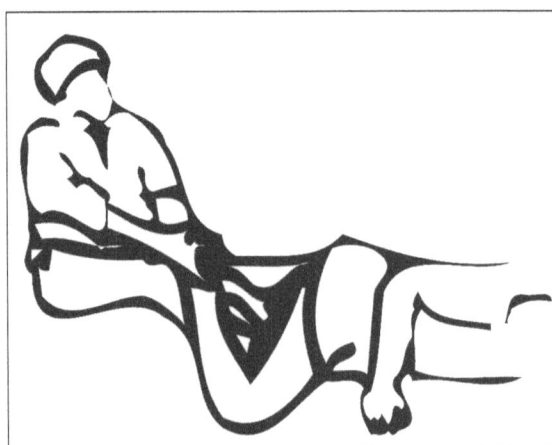

C. Release the lock and walk on the posterior aspect with both feet.

Sit up straight and allow the legs to do the work for you.

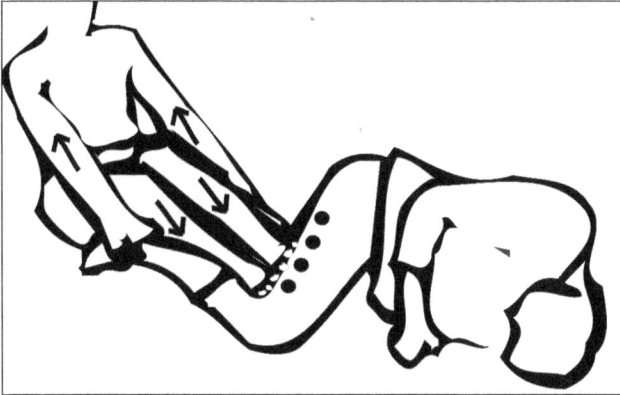

D. Lock the leg and ankle over both of your feet.
Slide up closer to your client and hook and pull the #1 outside line on the upper thigh. Still using the hooking technique walk the hands along the line.

Finish with soft fist percussion (Knocking) along the same lines.

If it is too dificult to reach over your knees then spread them wide and reach between them.

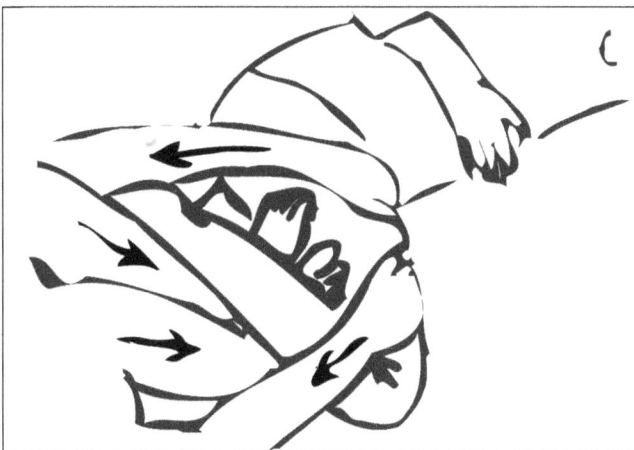

52. S.L.P. Superior Hip

52. S.L.P. Superior Hip

Warm up the hip area with palm pressure from the knee to the hip. Palm circle around the hip itself. Thumb press the #1 outside line to the hip and hold the last or topmost point (mid-Tensor fascialata).

Thumb press the #2 outside line of the upper leg to just below the hip, press and hold the top most point.

Thumb press the #3 outside line of the upper leg to just behind the hip bone and then press and hold the topmost point.

Press and hold each of these three hip points for five seconds.

Note: The points form a basic triangle with each point located no more than a thumbs-length apart.

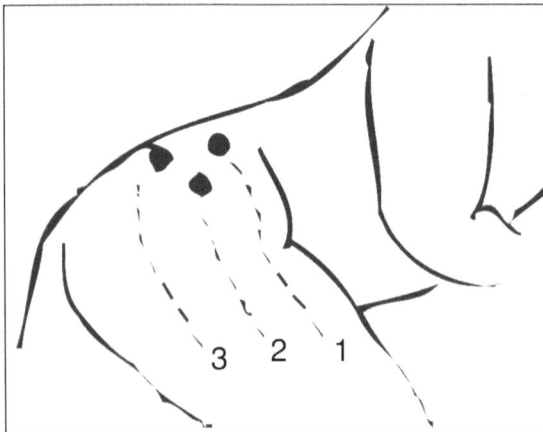

53. S.L.P. Superior Back Line

Warm up the back line with gentle palm pressure moving from the shoulder downward to the sacrum then back again.

Affects the sacrospinalis, quadratus lumborem, multifidi, rotatores, and latissimus dorsi muscles.

Palm walk in the same fashion.

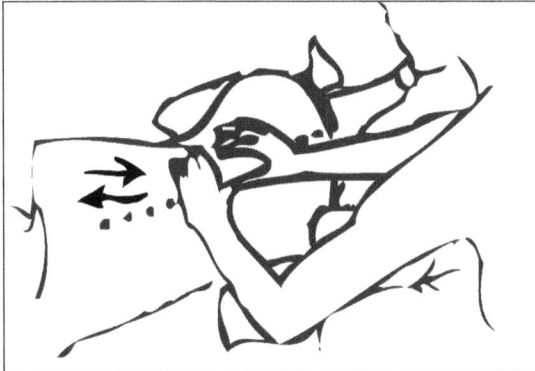

Begin at the sacrum and work upward to the shoulder with reinforced thumb technique then Thumb Walk down, returning to the sacrum.

Press and hold each of three points from the SI (Sacral Iliac) joint to the Superior aspect of the ischium two times.

Palm Press above the sacrospinalis then Palm Walk down again to finish.

1) **Warm-up the back...** PP, up, down
2) **PW, up, down**
3) **TP up, TW down**
4) **TP 3 Hip points**
5) **PP, up & down**
6) **PW, up & down**

54. S.L.P. Simultaneous Shoulder/Hip Rotation

Catch the shoulder in a finger cradle and lever over the waist with the elbow. Press each of three lower back points with the elbow by pulling on the shoulder while pressing with the point of the elbow. Work each point three times. (1, 2, 3, 2, 1)

Affects the rhomboids major and minor, sopraspinatus, medial and lower trapezius, and levator scapula muscles.

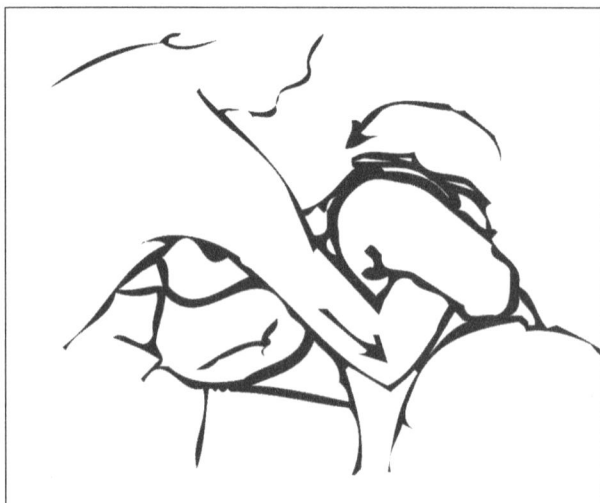

55. S.L.P. Superior Arm Raise & Press
A. Raise the superior arm straight up and support
it with your knee and hand.
   Stretch the arm in three positions over the head.
Position 1. Palm press at Axila (arm pit)
Position 2. Upper ribs
Position 3. Middle ribs

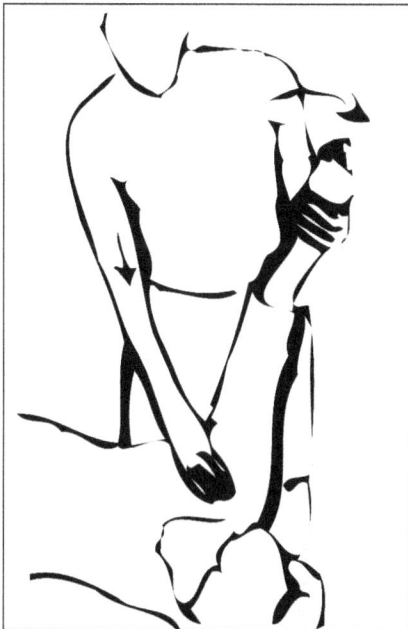

B. Continue stretching arm toward the back
over the leg in a lever-like motion. Palm press in
three positions.
Position 1. On the shoulder (Deltoid)
Position 2. The upper arm (Biceps)
Position 3. Mid-upper arm.

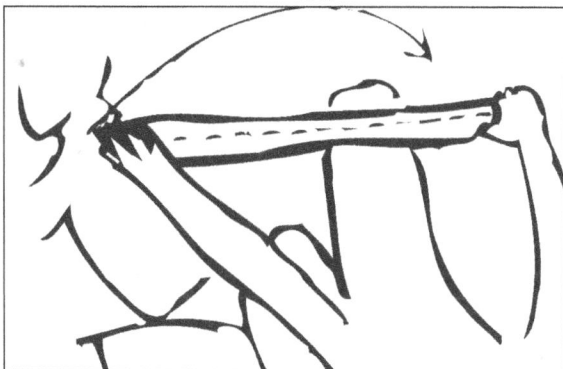

C. Palm Press from the shoulder area out to the
wrist then return to the shoulder.

56. S.L.P. Superior Lateral Arm Press
Warm up with Standard Palm Walk Procedure.

Thumb Walk from the back of the wrist up the center line of the lateral arm and then return to the wrist.

Palm Press from the wrist upward to the cap of the shoulder, then return to the wrist.

Affects the medial deltoid, bradioradialis muscles. The compression affects the musculature under the arm as well . By compressing the upper chest and abdomen this motion also works as a thoracic pump, moving fluids in the chest and stretching thoracic fasciae.

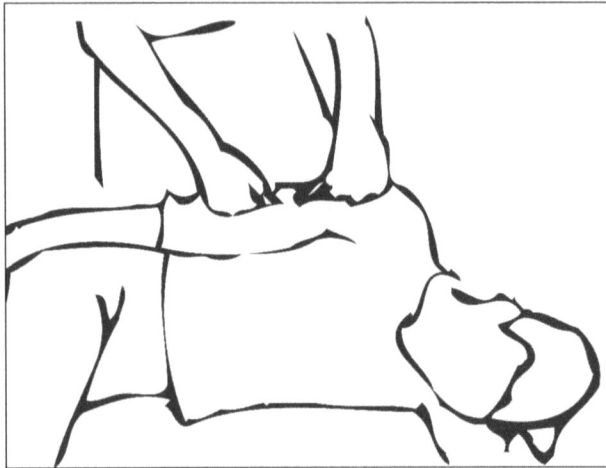

57. S.L.P. Hand Treatment
Warm up and stretch the hand thoroughly. Generally the Thai style hand treatment from the North is like that of the feet.

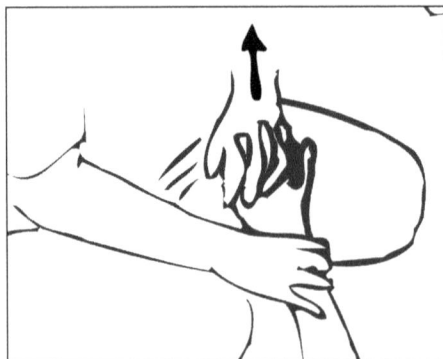

A. Six Palm Points (Posterior Hand)

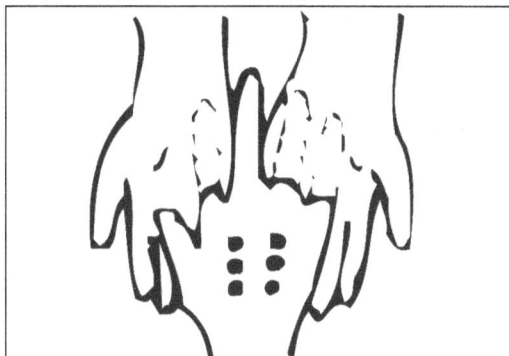

Essentially the same routine used in the supine position method.

Same as Step #41 on P. 79

B. Five Palm Lines (Posterior Hand) (Step 42)

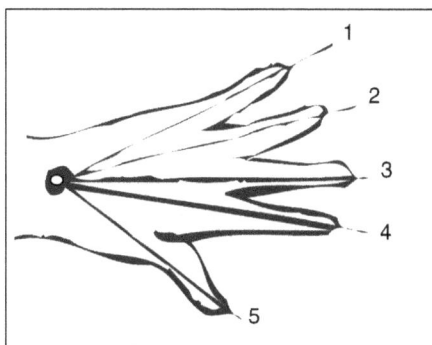

Same as Step #42 on P. 79

C. Four Lines (Anterior Hand) (Step 43)

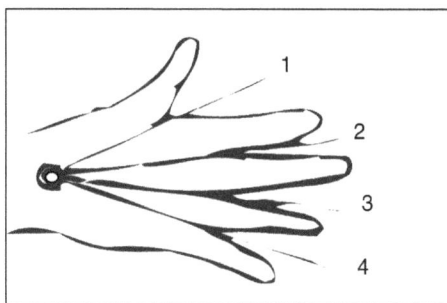

Same as Step #43 on P. 80

D. Rotate wrist and stretch fingers.

Same as Step #44 on P. 81

Interlock your fingers with those of your client while supporting their arm with the free hand. Rotate the wrist and hand several times in each direction.

Locking the fingers firmly pull and stretch the fingers three times.

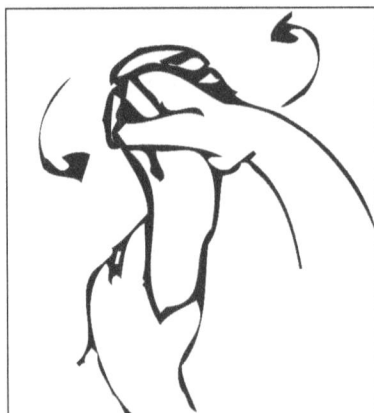

E. Pull the fingers.

Same as Step #45 on P. 82

Grasp each finger in turn. The joints of the fingers may pop or crack, however, this is not the sole intention. If the joint releases with an audible sound fine, if it does not, that is fine as well.

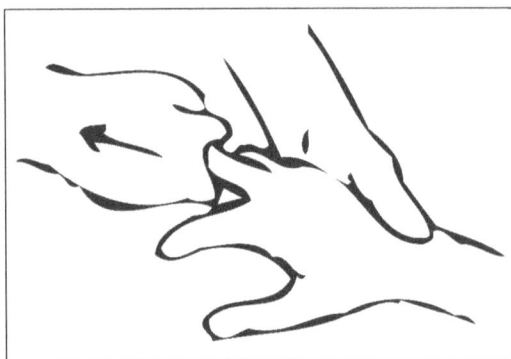

F. Palm Press and stretch the fingers. (Step 46)

Same as Step #46 on P. 83

After pulling the fingers, flip the fingers upward without turning the wrist. Hold the hand firmly and rub and stretch the entire palm surface between your thumbs.

Use the thumbs together and in opposition to create friction.

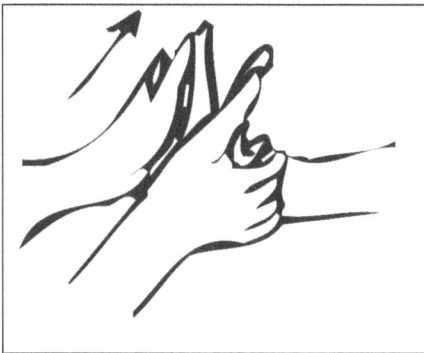

Make sure that you then stretch out each individual finger from bottom to the tip, one at a time. Be careful not to over stretch in this position as you have a lot of leverage against any individual finger.

58. S.L.P. Bent Arm Press

Raise the arm to the ear and invert the hand on to the side of the client's head.

A. Tiger Hand, squeeze and pull both sides of the arm from base to elbow 3X.

B. Press the elbow and hip in opposite directions.

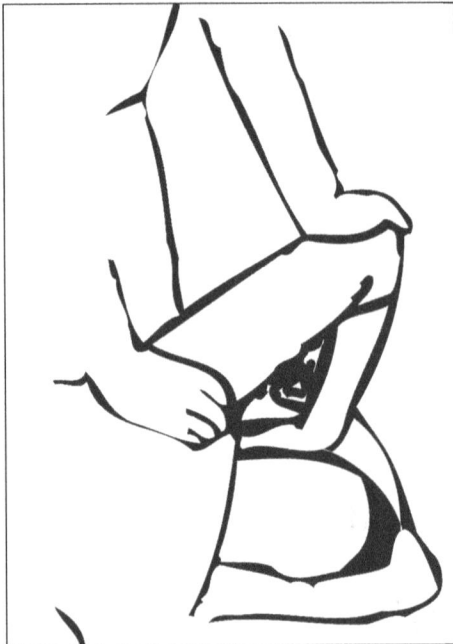

C. While pressing on the elbow, pull three points on the posterior upper arm with the opposite hand.

59. S.L.P. Spinal Rotation and Stretch
A. From the side lying position, brace the superior
knee with the lower hand and move the client's arm
away from the body 90°. Now, press the shoulder on
the same side toward the mat as far as possible,
within the tolerance of the client. It is very normal to
hear one or a series of loud "pops" or "cracks" as this
range of motion exercise is done. It is not the
purpose of this movement to cause the back to crack.
Rather, it is a stretch and rotation of the spine, as well
as the muscles and nerves around the spine. This
primarily facilitates the flow of Chi (prana) through
the bladder channel and related Sen. Any specific
vertebral motion is incidental to the stretch.

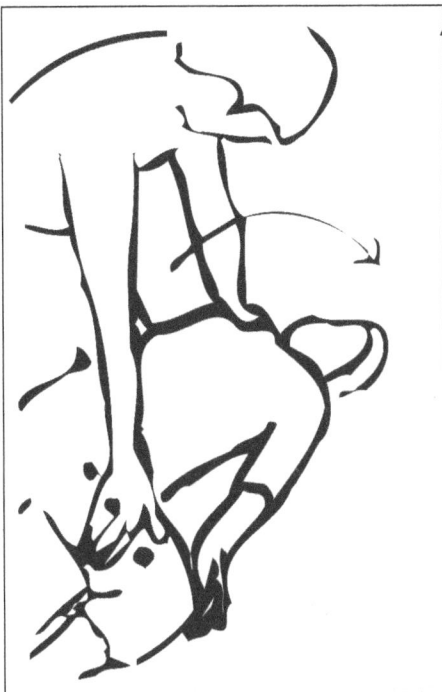

B. With the lower hand work with palm pressure
three points on the superior lateral leg.
1. Lower outer thigh
2. Mid lateral thigh
3. Upper lateral thigh

104

60. S.L.P. Psoas Stretch

Dhanurasana

The Bow Pose

A. The working knee is raised to massage the superior muscles along the spine just above the waist. Raise and support the leg by cradling the knee and support the shoulder with the upper arm. Pull the shoulder and the supported leg at the same time while applying knee pressure to each of three low back points. (1,2,1) Only press points above the spine.

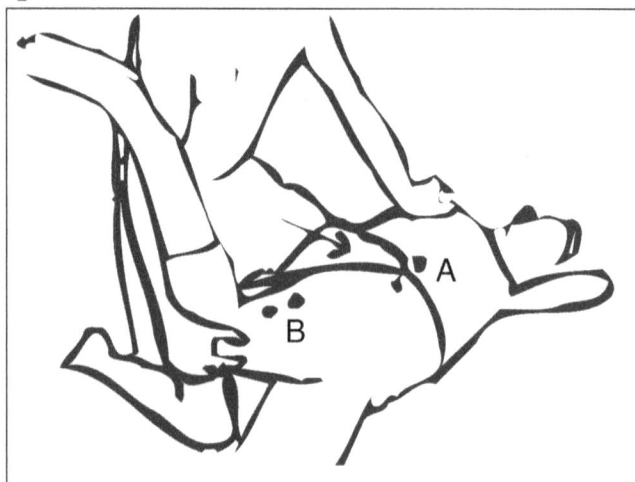

B. Change knees and work three points on the supported leg.
1. Mid-gluteal
2. Upper thigh
3. Mid thigh
    Now release the shoulder and use the free hand to Palm Walk the #1 outside line of the upper leg. Finish with percussion techniques along the same line.

61. S.L.P. Spinal Rotation and Lift
Stand below the bent superior leg, straddling the
straight leg. Grasp the inferior wrist and hand firmly
and bend your knees in preparation for lifting. Pull
up three times. Each time release slowly being
careful not to drop your client!

    Finish with some nice palm circles along the
spine to relax.

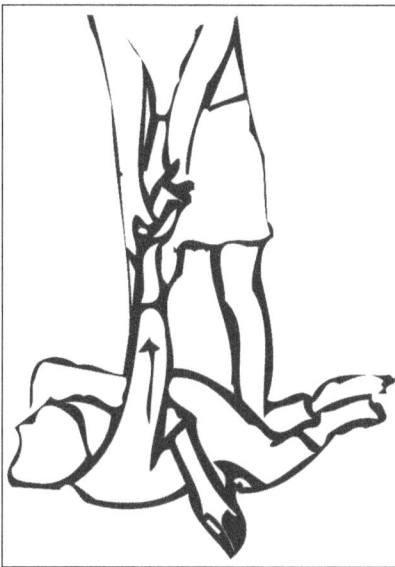

62. S.L.P. Standing Psoas Pull Up
A. Grasp the superior hand and the inferior ankle,
fix the working foot above the spine. Pull hand and
ankle (a) while using foot pressure to work three
 points along superior spine. The attitude should be
easy and smooth. The therapist should stand erect
and strive to be sensitive while pulling.

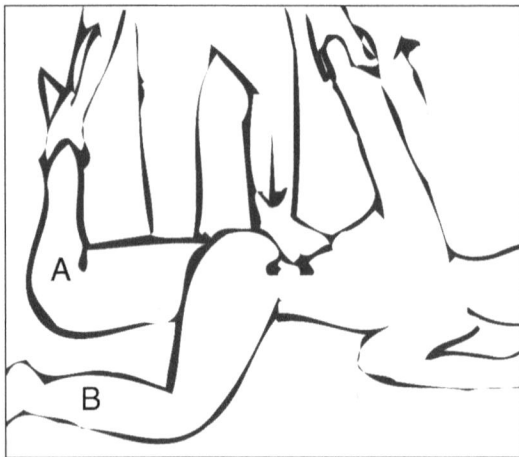

B. Release ankle (a) and pick up ankle (b) and
repeat procedure.

Roll the client over to the oposite side and repeat steps #49 through #62

P. 90 through P. 106

Do the Warm Up again. Relax the feet and the legs with Palm Walking from the ankles up to the hips, returning to the ankles and feet.
Step 32 x 3 Crossed Leg Pull up
Step 33 x 1 Seated Shoulder Press

Synopsis: Side Lying Position

63. With the client face down, warm up with Palm Walking from the bottoms of the feet to the gluteal area. Use a soft hand and relaxing method as you move up and down the leg.

Stand facing the client's back and walk on the soles of the feet gently. Begin initially with pressure from the ball of your foot and once you have thoroughly covered the whole foot, turn around and work the foot with your heels. Walk softly and gently, allow your weight to be light and remember your breath. Finish the walking by returning once again to the ball of your foot.

Kneel down placing your knees gently on the soles of your client's feet and Palm Walk again up and down the legs.

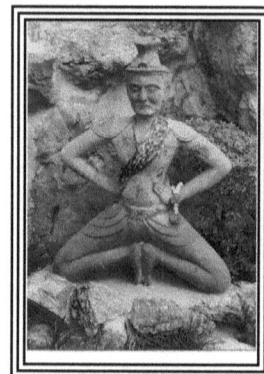

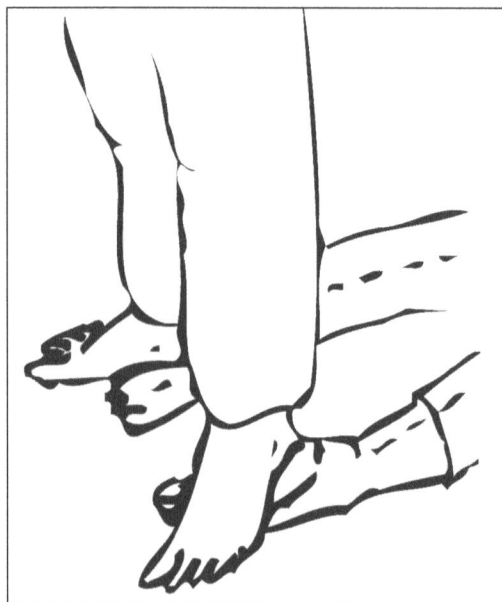

(Men, right; Women, left)

It may be helpfull when working especially with women to prop the chest up slightly with a pillow.. The client should turn their head comfortably to the side.

64. Foot Treatment

Note: See Supine foot routine for illistrations.

Raise the foot and support it securely by stepping forward with one knee and laying the foot over your thigh.

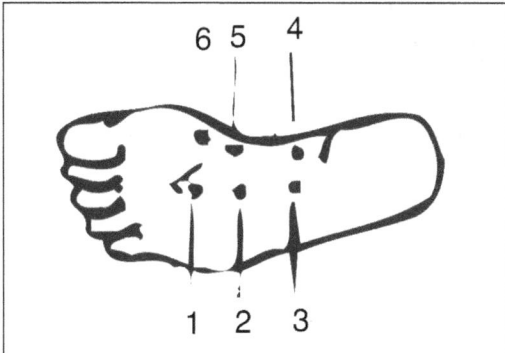

A. Six points with elbow pressures
B. Elbow/forearm rolling and knocking
C. Five lines with thumb pressure
D. Thumb walk on entire foot
E. Press foot forward and work four lines
F. Palm press them work five arch points
G. Ankle Rotations 5 x each way
H. Twist the foot inside and outside
I. Pull the toes

9 Steps Foot Routine
General reflexology

1) 6 Pts.
2) Forearm Roll
3) 5 Lines
4) TP
5) 4 Lines
6) 5 Arch Pts.
7) Rotate Ankle
8) Twist foot
9) Pull Toes

65. Ankle Rotation with the Supported Forearm

Reach over the bottom of the foot and grasp the heel. Lay the forearm lengthwise along the foot. Support the top of the foot with your free hand and rotate the foot against this platform of your arms. Widen the radius of your circle maintaining a horizontal plane of movement with your arms.

Press the foot as far forward as you comfortably can go and then return.

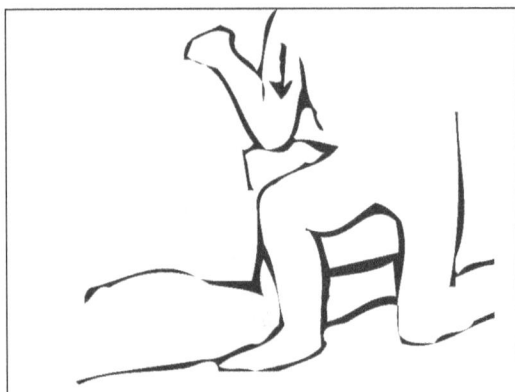

Change feet and repeat step #64 & 65. on the opposite foot.

66. Inverted V Press (Downward Dog)

(Bhekasana)

Palm walk with the breath up, down up. Stop at the top and deepen the posture. Keep your head and neck relaxed throughout.

Begin at the feet and palm walk up and down the back of the legs. Work this line again Thumb Walking simultaneously up both legs. Upon reaching the gluteal area place the palms firmly below the buttocks with the fingertips pointing away from the center line. Push up and raise your body into the Dog pose or inverted V shape. Your head should be between your arms and your feet, planted a foot width apart, should be flat. The heels are pressed to the floor. Relax and breathe as you hold this position for one to five minutes. Bend your arms and lower your knees to release pressure gradually. Palm walk returning to the feet.

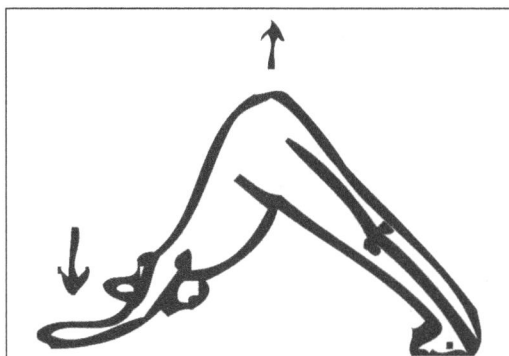

67. Prone Planar Toe Press

Raise and Palm Press the toes toward the buttocks in line with the legs. Press three times soft, firm then soft again.

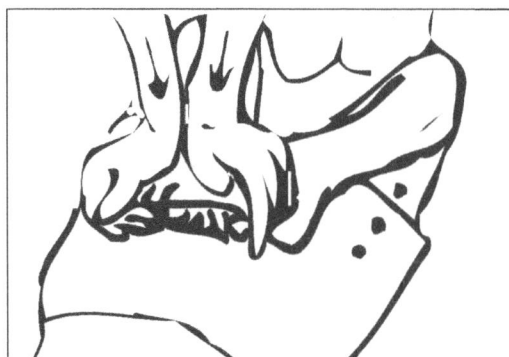

68. Prone Heel Press
Use the Supported Forearm Technique demonstrated in Step #65 working both feet simultaneously.

Press both heels into the bottom three times, soft, firm and soft again.

(Bent Knee Position)

NOTE: Affects the gluteus maximus, tensor fascial latae, iliotibial band, adductor magnus, gastrocnemius, soleus, peroneus longus, tibialis anterior.

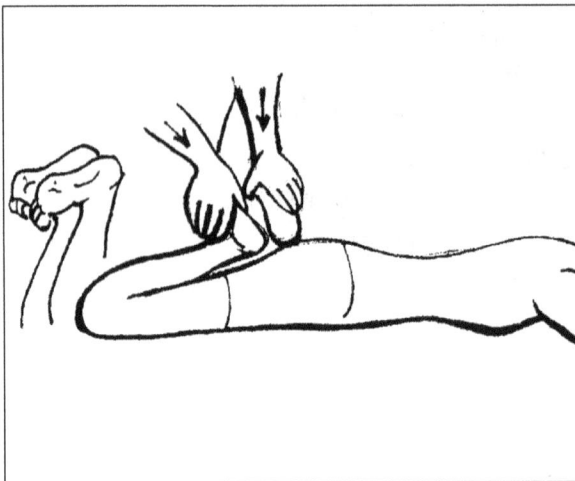

69. Prone Crossed Toe Press
Cross the raised feet at the balls and press to the buttocks. Change and repeat.It is useful to hold both feet crossed securely with one hand while working the #1 outside line of the lower leg with thumb pressure from the ankle to the knee.

(Frog Pose)

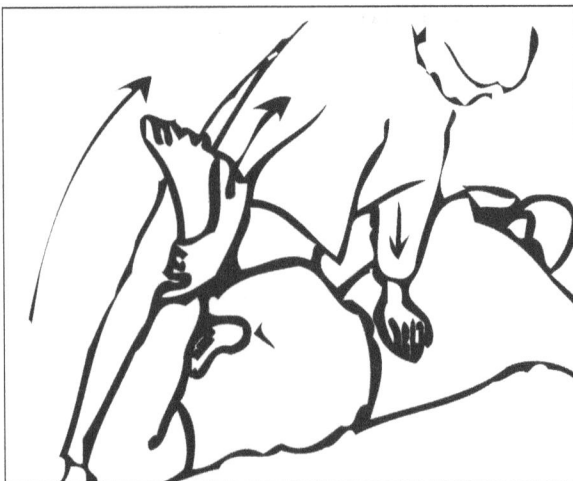

70. Prone Posterior Lateral Leg

Fold the leg inward so the foot comes to a position over the posterior of the opposite knee. Palm Press on the ankle while working 3 points on the upper bent leg with palm pressure. (1, 2, 3, 2, 1)

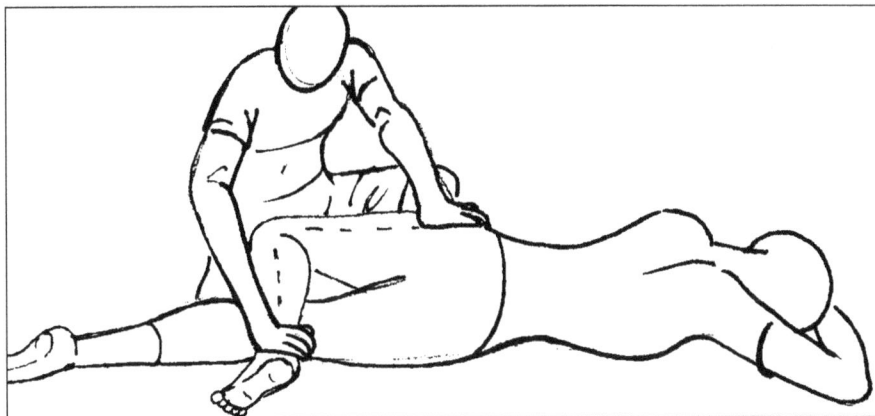

71. Folding the Leg

Fold the straight leg over the foot and support the ankle. Press and lever the ankle inward over the trapped foot while working three points on the outer thigh of the upper leg (1, 2, 3, 2, 1).

Fold left over right for women and right over left for men.

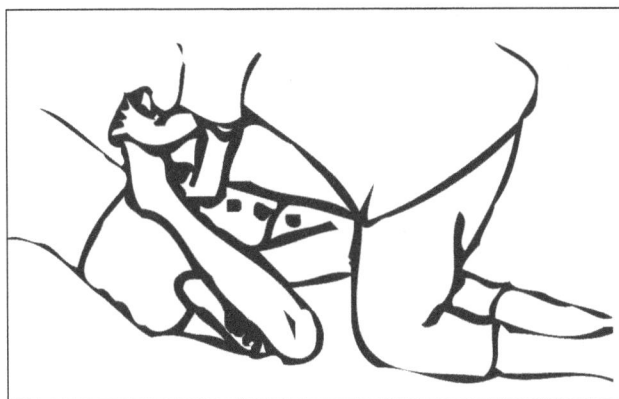

72. Folding the Leg with Knee Pressure
Move to a position kneeling beside the client facing the feet. Kneel gently on the side of the lower back closest to you (L5 area). Grasp the ankle with one hand and lift the knee with the other. Massage three points on the lower back while lifting and stretching (1,2,3,2,1)

In this position do not actually press with the knee. The idea is really more to lightly place the knee in the appropriate position and then lift into the stationary knee. Avoid leaning on the back with too much pressure. Support your bodyweight with the knee remaining on the floor.

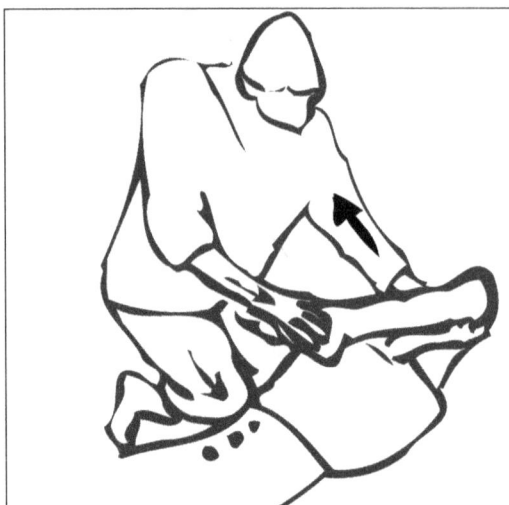

73. Folding the Leg with Palm Pressure
In the kneeling position reach across the body with the upper hand and work the same three points used in Step #72 with Palm Pressure. Lift and stretch by pulling the raised ankle as you do so. It is okay to lift at the knee as well.

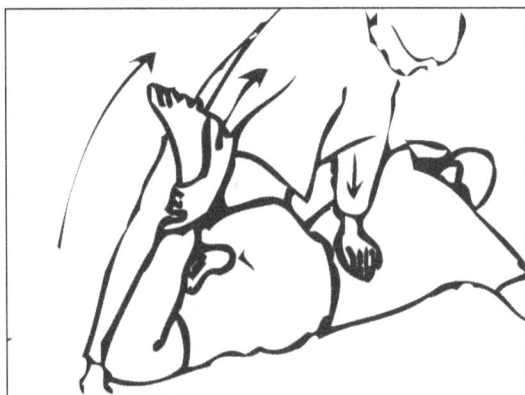

Change sides and repeat steps #70 through #73

74. Prone Lower Back/Hip and Leg—Seated Position

5 Steps:
1) Stretch
2) Elbow Low Back/ SI
3) Rolling Forearm
- Hip to Shoulder
- Glut and Thigh
- Leg to calf
4) Hitting
5) Press Out 3X

Lift the whole leg (left/woman) and slide under the leg and upper thigh. Sit Thai Style with both of your legs turned and folded to the side nearest the client's feet.

The client's leg should be stretched out straight across your lap.

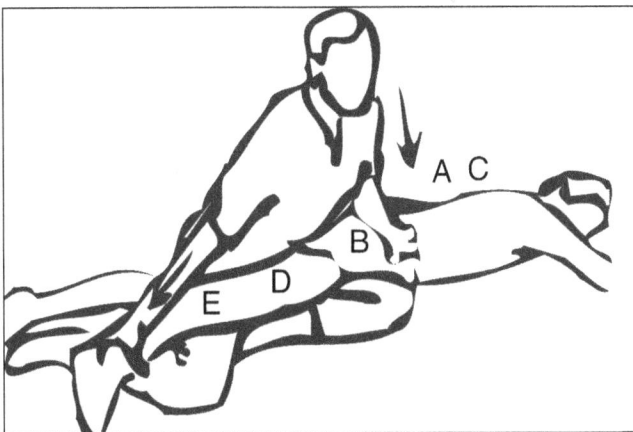

A. Stretch hip and lower leg to the foot with the hand and the forearm.
B. Press for 10 counts at L5 hip joint with elbow/forearm pressure.
C. Massage with rolling forearm technique from the hip to the shoulder area three times. Hold the waist point again for 10 counts.
D. Massage with Rolling Forearm Technique the posterior hip glut and thigh one time.
E. Continue by changing arms rolling down the back of the leg including the calf area.
F. Use Percussion and Hacking Technique on the back of the hip/gluteal area.
G. Begin at the section of the upper leg on your lap and press out both forearms simultaneously - moving them away from each other three times.

Change sides and repeat step #74 on the opposite side.

75. Sit on Feet/Press with Palm
Fold the feet upward together to make a seat or
stool and facing the clients head sit firmly on them.
Your feet are forward enough to create a stable
platform for you to work.

(Bhujangasana)

A. Palm Press up and down the spine in a
bilateral fashion. Then palm walk up/down to relax.

A. PP up and down,
PW up and down.

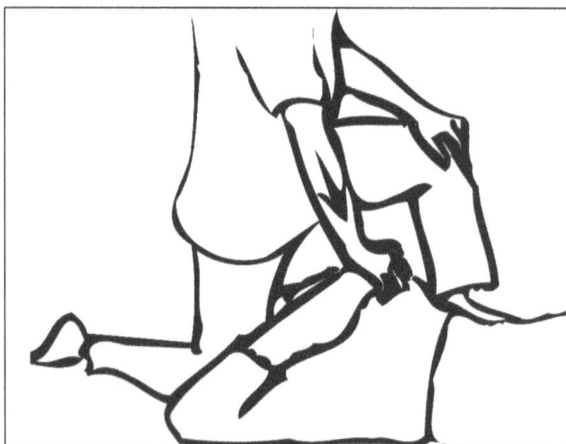

B. Work bilateral points alongside the back from
sacrum to the shoulders then Thumb Walk down.

B. TP up
TW down

TP up
TW down

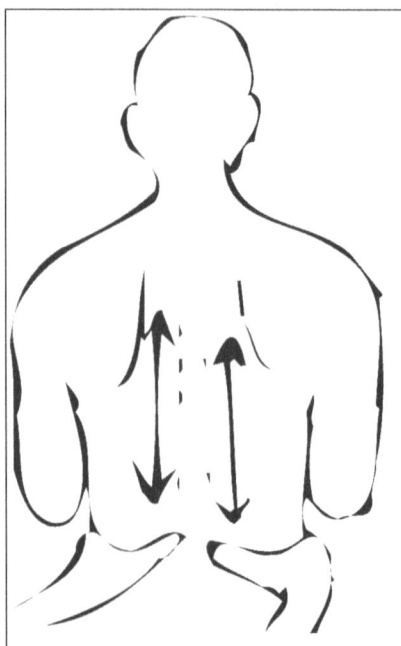

C. Thumb Press 3 hip points on the posterior hip
(1,2,3,2,1) and then massage the bilateral points
again to the upper shoulder.

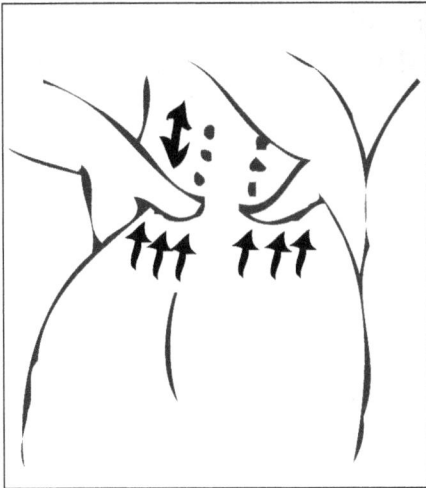

TP out & back
TP up

D. Hold and press the bilateral points at C7 for
five counts then the apex point at the top of the
spine for five counts. Then Palm Walk down to the
hip area.

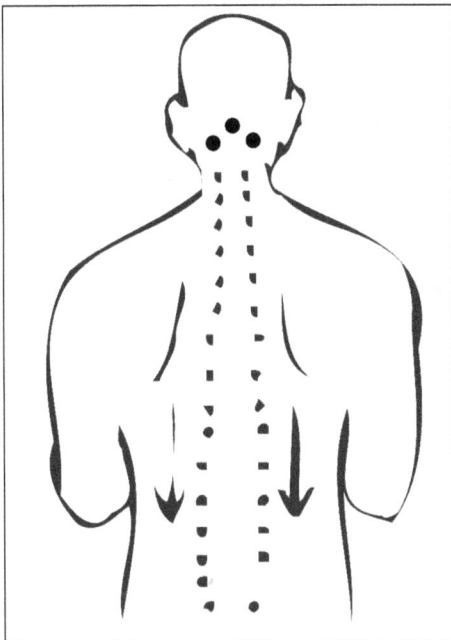

TP pts. #1 & 2
PW down

76. The Seated Cobra
Raise both arms up and back onto your thighs.

A. First grasp the trapezium area and pull, shifting you weight away from the shoulders just until the upper body begins to lift and hold five counts.

A) Trapesious (top of shoulder)

B) Shoulder (outside shoulder on the Deltoid muscle)

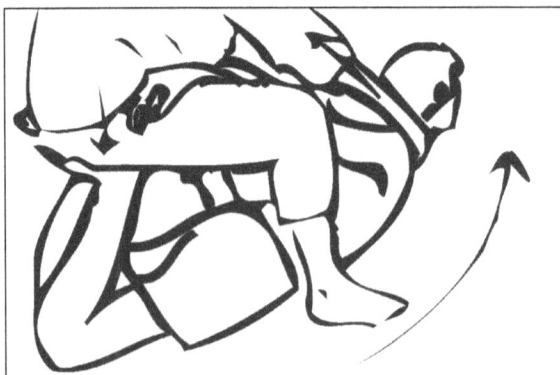

B. Reach under the shoulder and lift three times.

77. Half Kneeling Cobra
Kneeling with a raised leg across the client bring their arm up and on top of your knee/thigh. Palm Press around the shoulder blade. Thumb Press around the shoulder blade while lifting the shoulder. Use a gentle rocking motion as you simultaneously lift and Thumb Press.

Do both Sides!

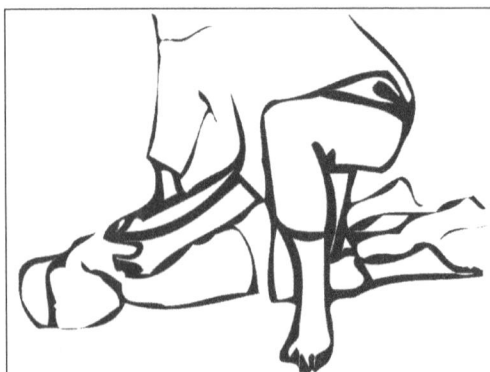

Change sides and repeat step #77

78. The Cobra Stretch
Palm Press and Palm Walk up to the shoulder then down to the waist. Palm Walk again up the sides of the spine then out to the shoulders and down the arms to the triceps when you reach the hands. Kneeling position on the buttocks, grasp both wrists individually with both hands and pull the arms backwards, raising the client's body up and back. It is helpful if the client holds onto your wrists as well. Hold the position for five counts each of three times.
Position 1. Kneeling on the gluteal
Position 2. Hip and thigh
Position 3. Upper thigh
Next rotate the client's torso to one side while lifting, then rotate to the opposite side. Slowly return to the center and release.

Palm pressure walking from the hands, up the arms to the shoulder. Move down the back all the way down the legs finishing with the feet and ankle.

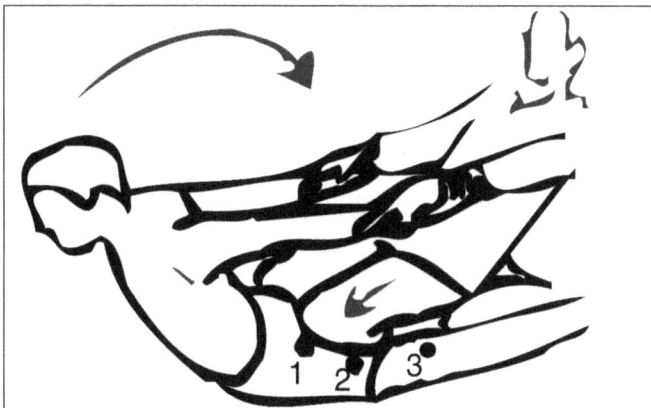

79. Wheelbarrow

Raise both ankles like lifting the handles of a wheelbarrow and walk forward. Stabilize the foot on the sacrum using the heel or the ball of the foot. Use the heel to press three points on the lower back (1, 2, 1). Change feet and repeat the procedure on the opposite side. Now turn the foot 90° and work both sides of the lower back. The arch of your foot should rest over the spinous process of the spine without undo pressure. (1, 2, 1)

This is another position where you lift into the pressure as opposed to actually stepping down to create or generate pressure.

Remember no direct pressure on the spinal vertebrae!

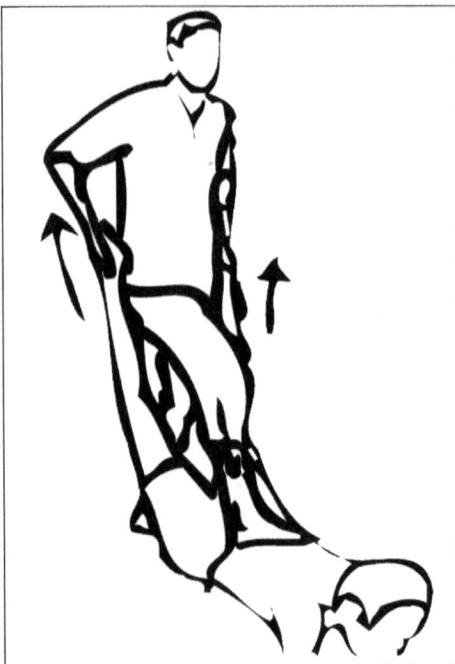

80. Standing and Lifting
Women should stand on the left, men on the right.

A. Pick up the hand closest to you and the opposite ankle. Place a heel on the low back point closest to the L5 Junction. Pull both the ankle an the hand to apply pressure.

B. Pick up the hand and ankle on the same side and repeat.

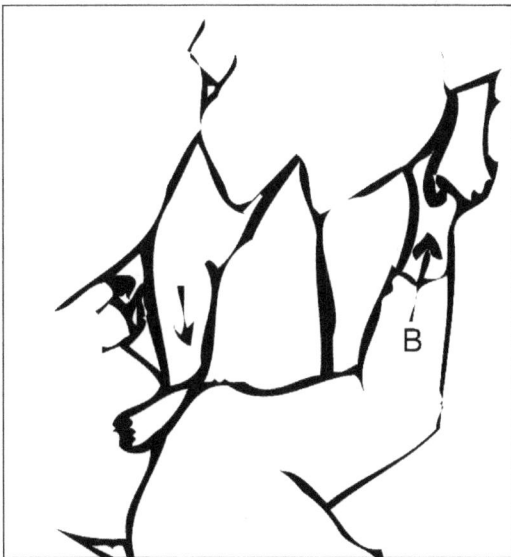

Change sides and repeat step #80

81. Cross Stretching with Palms

In the kneeling position beside the client place the palms at opposite points of the torso. One hand is placed on the posterior shoulder and the other on the hip. The hands should be on opposite sides of the spine. Lean on the hands and stretch, imparting a slight rotation. Release and move the upper hand caudally or toward the hip and repeat.

Work methodically in one hand width spacing down to the hip. Change hands and begin again at the shoulder and hip.

Relax the whole back with gentle palm circles.

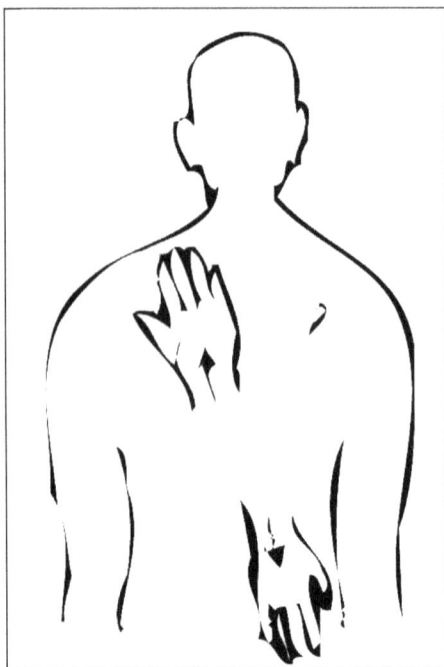

Synopsis: Prone Position

82. Seated Position Shoulder Press (Step #33)
Move in close to stand immediately behind your client. Use your legs to give the client who is in a relaxed seated position some support. Apply palm #110 pressure on three points moving outward from the base of the neck to the shoulder. The fingers of the hand are pointing toward the client's back moving out and are turned forward toward the chest while returning to the neck area again.

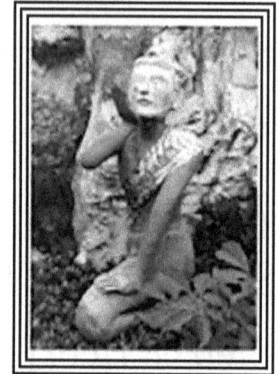

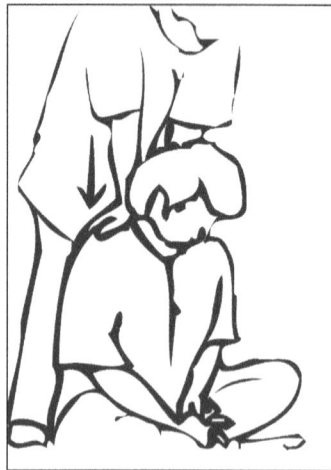

Work the points in sequence:
1, 2, 3, 2, 1

83. Seated Position Thumb Press
Use Thumb pressure to work four or five points outward and back pressing from the base of the neck to the shoulder. Massage the points in a bilateral fashion.

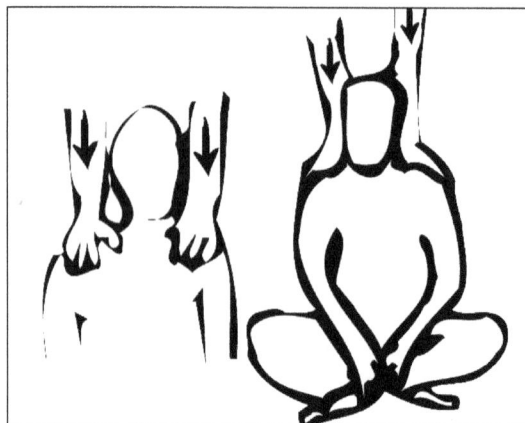

Work the points in sequence:
1, 2, 3, 4, 5, 4, 3, 2, 1

84. Relaxing the Back in Seated Position
In a kneeling position behind the client use Thumb Pressure to lightly work the bilateral neck points down to and outward along the tops of the shoulders.

Palm press down the sides of the spine and Palm Walk returning to the neck.

Thumb walk down the sides of the spine. Thumb press outward over the posterior crest of the hips and then finish by Thumb Walking upward along the sides of the spine again returning to the shoulder area.

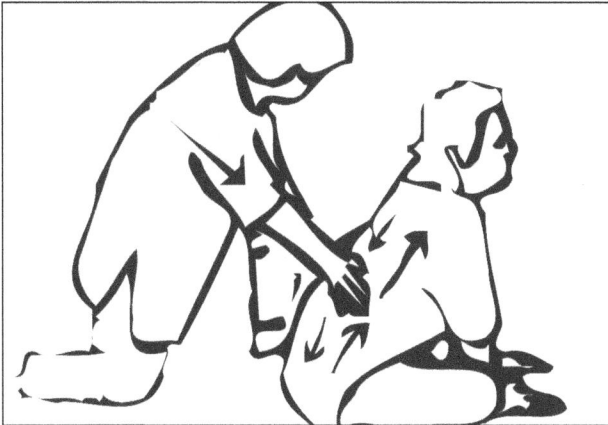

Relaxing the Back

TP Up/Down neck
TP out/ back shoulder
PP down
PW up
TW down
TP out/back Hips
TW up to shoulder/neck

85. Seated Bilateral Neck Points
Lightly grasp the sides of the client's neck while you work 5 points on both sides of the cervical spine to the base of the head or cranium. Move downward working the points again.

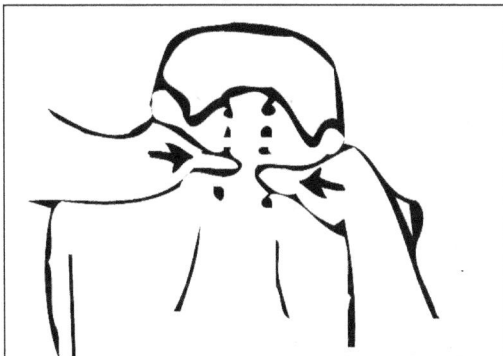

86. Seated Position Posterior Medial Scapula

Bring the arm and the hand located on the same side as the scapula you wish to work around behind the back. Kneel into the palm of the hand to secure it. Reach around with the outside hand and pull the shoulder posteriorly while massaging the medial area of the scapula with thumb pressure.

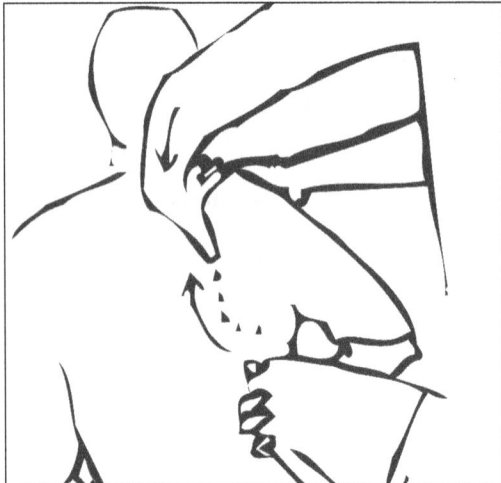

87. Seated Position Elbow Press

Kneeling behind the client and supporting them upright with the side of your knee, pull their hand up and over behind their head. You should be facing at a right angle to your client. Grasp their hand firmly with your inside arm and lever downward onto the top of the shoulder working three points (1, 2, 3, 2, 1). If you wish you may add additional support to the arm being massaged with your outside hand.

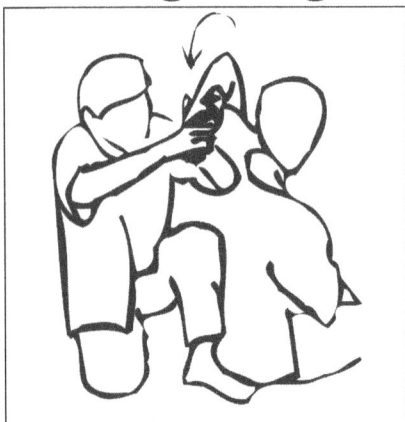

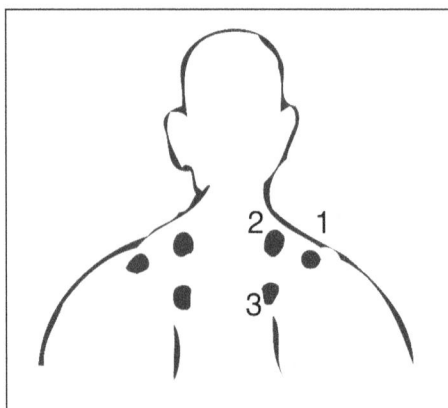

88. Seated Posterior Upper Arm

Raise and bend the arm you wish to massage up and bend the arm over backwards placing the **palm of that hand on the back**.

Kneeling behind and facing into the client, support the elbow with your inside hand. Hook and pull the upper posterior line of the triceps with finger pressure and then finish by knocking.

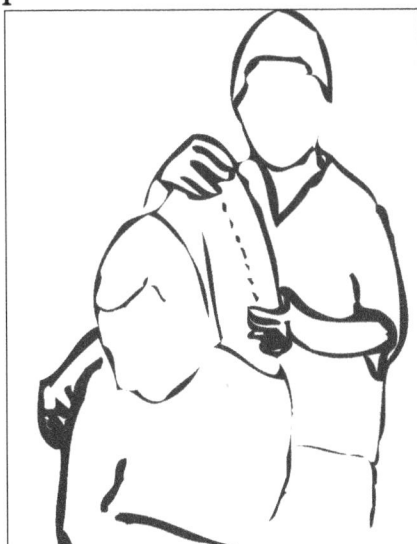

89. Seated Forearm Wedge and Roll

Lean forward and place both forearms alongside one another, clasping the hands together. Use the inside forearm to lever the neck and the head to one side as you forearm roll out and back on top of the shoulder.

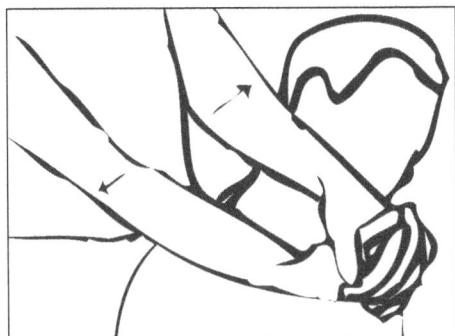

Change sides and repeat steps #86 through #89

90. Seated Posterior Cervical with Tiger Hand and Vise-Like Thumb

Relax the client's neck by gentle squeezing with the Tiger Hand Technique. Move the thumb and the fingers of the hand in gentle circles. This action soothes and comforts.

Lock the fingers and invert the hands into the Vise-like Thumb position. This technique is the same one as used in Sao Nong or Step #17B.

Squeeze five points bilaterally; two at a time.

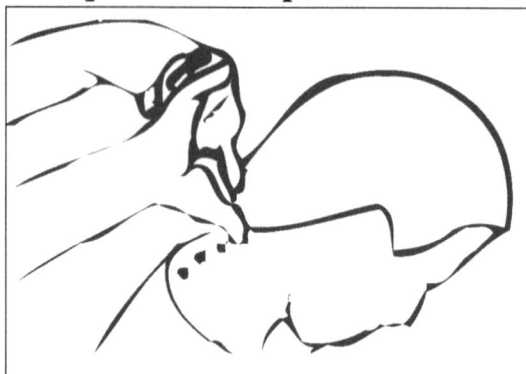

91. Seated Cranial Base Points

Begin by relaxing the base area of the cranium with bilateral thumb circles.

Next press and hold the point located at the midmont area of the occiput for five seconds and release slowly. Then hold the next point out bilaterally for five seconds and release slowly as well.

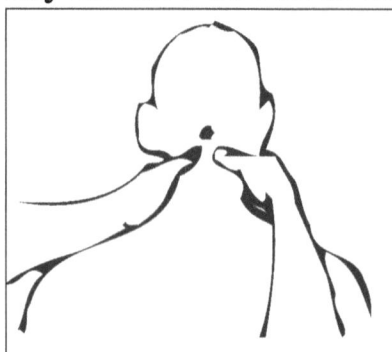

92. Seated Posterior Cranial Points

Reach around and support the forehead with one hand and press the points around the base of the cranium with thumb pressure. Begin from the center and work outward.

Return to the center and Thumb Press up the center line of the back of the head. As you reach the top, stand up in order to work. Hold the crown point equated with the Sahasara Chakra for five seconds and then release slowly. Use Reinforced Thumb pressure from the crown point to the hairline. Thumb Walk back to the crown point.

Use gentle shampoo technique with all of the fingers relaxing the head and scalp in general.

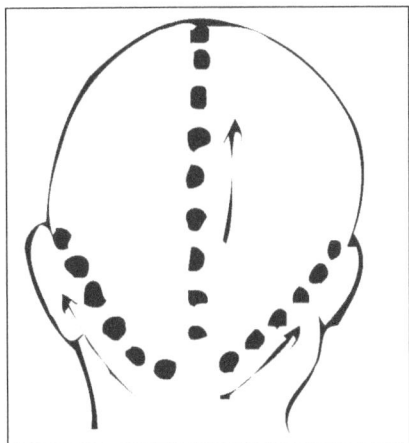

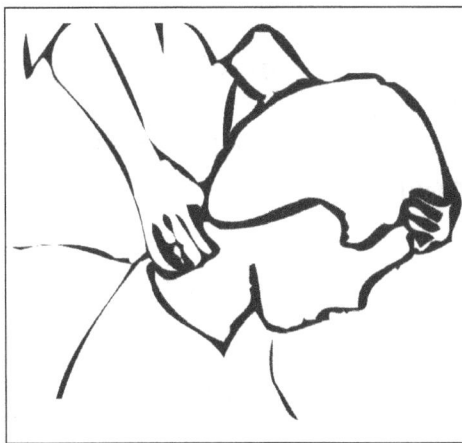

93. Seated Facial Treatment

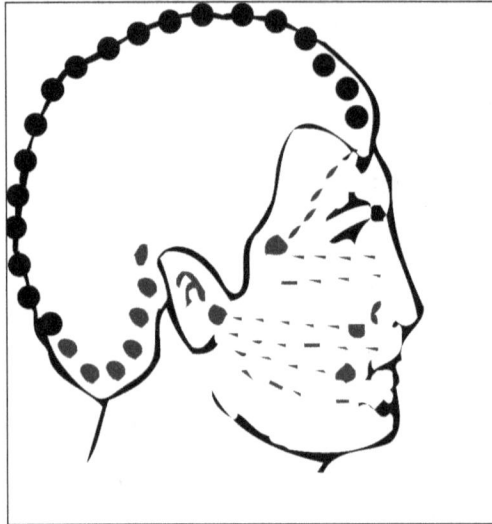

Move to a seated or kneeling position in front of the client.
1. Massage around the hairline, using thumb pressure, three times.
2. With the thumb, press out each line one time:
    a. Mid-forehead
    b. Eyebrow
    c. Under eyes
    d. Maxilla
    e. Mid-chin
3. Press the ears closed and hold for five seconds, release quickly.

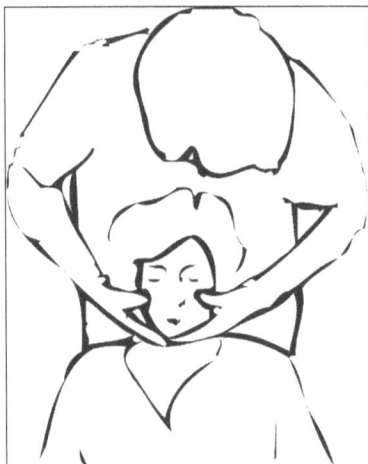

94.Seated Namaskar Mudra

While in the kneeling position behind the client and your hands in the traditional "Wai" position; roll with both forearms on top of the shoulders. Hold the client's head between your hands and slowly pull and tilt the head as far back as possible without straining. Move smoothly and return smoothly so that the client is relaxed and confident. Once back in the center position press with the elbow three points (1, 2, 3, 2, 1) Shoulder and Head Points.

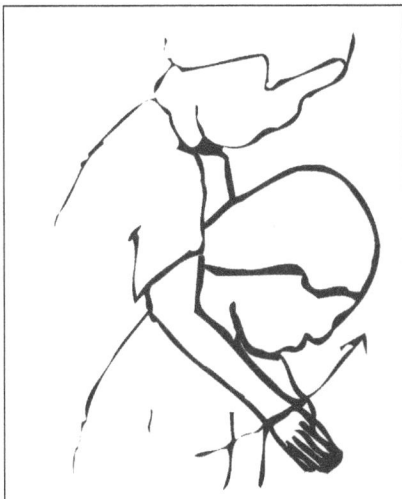

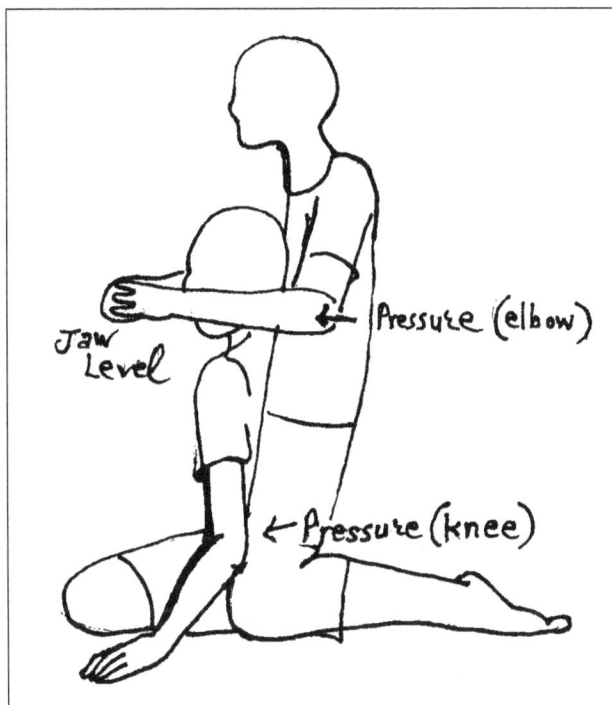

Shoulder and Head Points

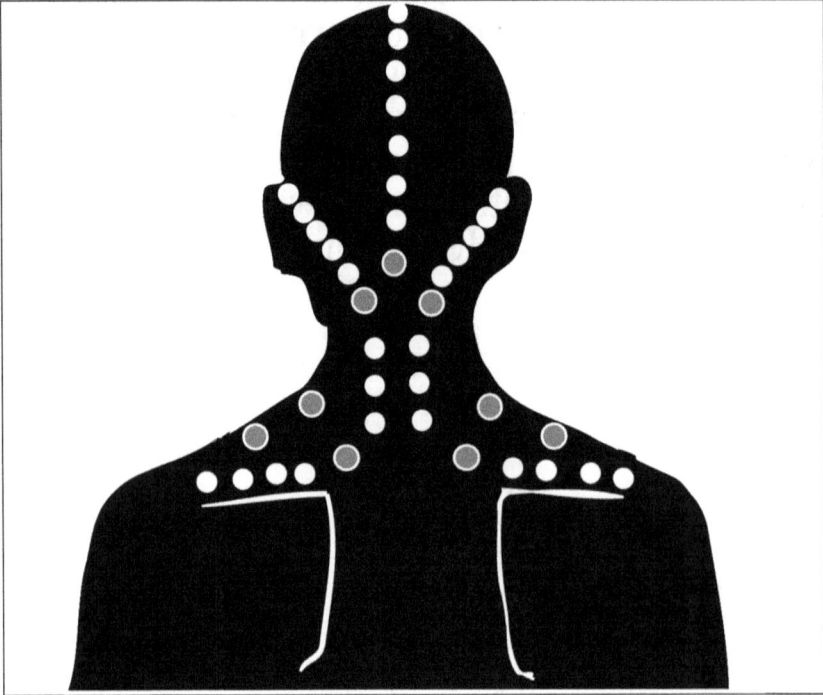

95. Reinforced Upper Torso Rotation With the hands of the client interlocked and clasped firmly behind the head, the therapist, in a kneeling position, reaches up and under the arms to grasp the forearms in a firm grip. The therapist will then brace the knee opposite the direction of rotation and once in the position twist and stretch as far as possible. Without altering the hand position, the therapist changes sides and repeats the procedure.

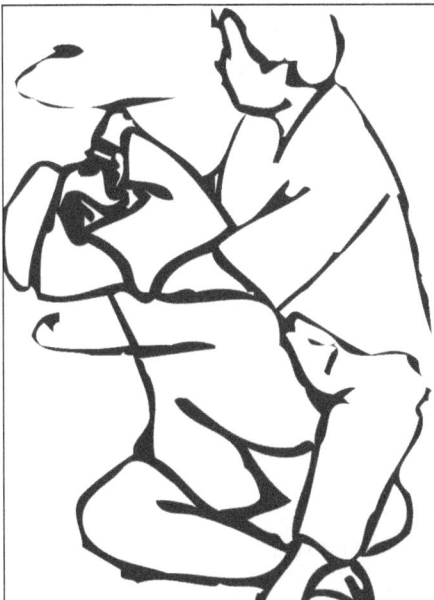

To finish press the upper torso of the client forward three times, stretching the lower back. It is extremely important to consider the comfort and range of motion of the client. Always work within the tolerance of the client and never force any movement. Go slow and develop or move into new range of motion with care and consideration.

96. Spinal Push While still holding the arms braced behind the head, raise both of your knees together to about T-12 and pull the client backwards on to the knees. Release and raise the knees an repeat. Do this three times, then finish the movement at the original position.

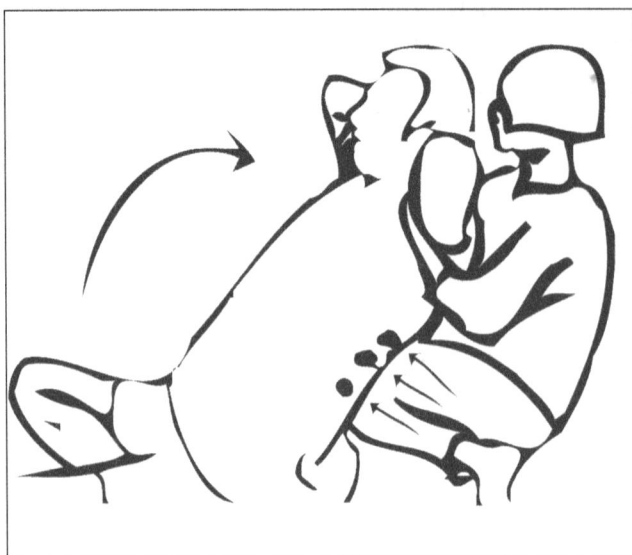

97. Spinal Push with Straight Arms
In a seated position behind your client, place the balls of your feet against the lower back. Grasp both of the client's arms pulling them to the rear.

Pull the arms gently and simultaneously press with the feet. Work three points to just below the bottom of the shoulders.

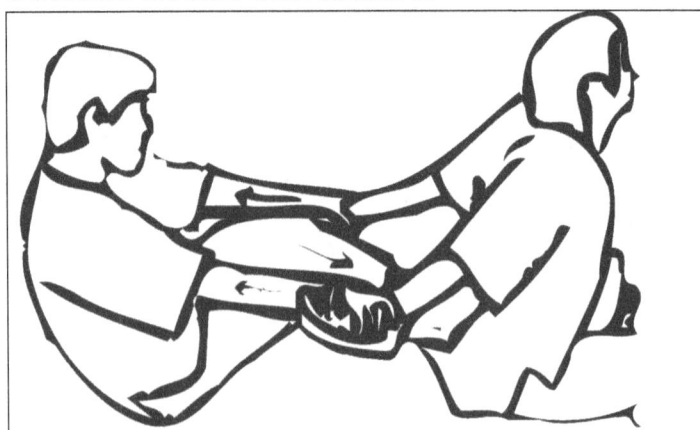

98. Spinal Push with Crossed Arms
Basically the same as step #96 or Spinal Push except that you cross the client's arms over each other and pull the hands to the rear as you press inward with the knees. Again, work three points. (1, 2, 3, 2, 1)

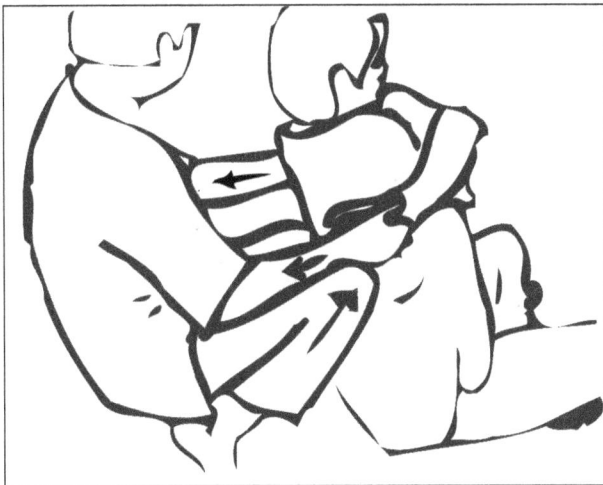

99. Hitting the Back
Kneeling behind the client, join the hands together in the Two Hand Hacking Position, and beginning at the neck and the shoulder area work out and down over the whole back. Repeat this over the back three times and then brush out to finish.

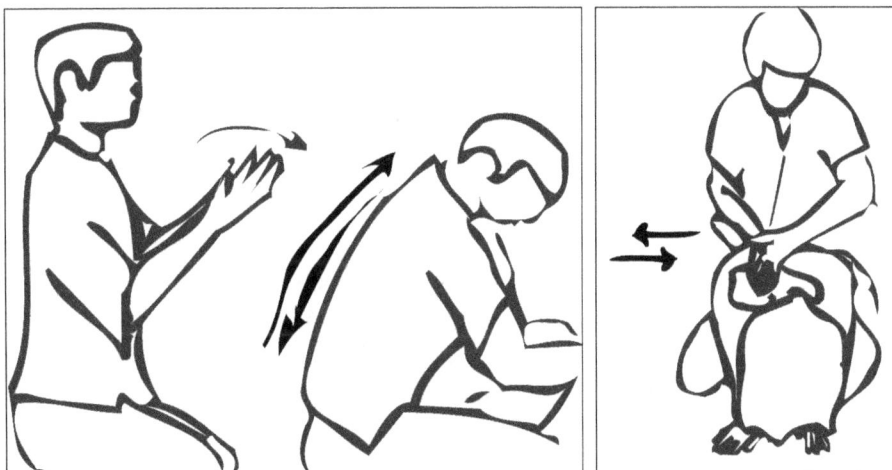

Synopsis: Seated Position

Relax the Back:
TP Neck up/down
TP Shoulder
  out/ back
PP down
PW up
TW down
TP out/ back
  (hip points)
TW up to neck

Change sides and repeat steps #86 through #89

Brush Out... Finnish

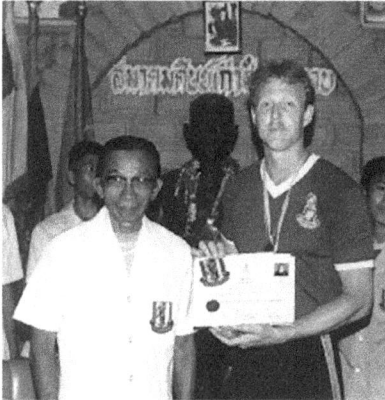

Mr. James, receiving his teaching certificate from Phaa Khruu Samaii Mesamarn of The Buddhai Swan Institute, Nongkam Thailand, 1986.

About the Author

Nuad Boran Master 2018Nuad Boran Master 2018Aachan, Anthony B. James CMT, ND(T), MD(AM), OMD, DPH(h.c.), RAAP stands out as the second non-ethnic Thai to be formally certified and recognized as a Khruu or teacher of traditional Thai martial and healing arts. Dr. James is the first United States instructor to receive recognition in Traditional Thai Medical Massage by both US and agencies in Thailand. First to be recognized by American Oriental Bodywork Therapists Association (AOBTA , Instructor Certificate #32) and the Association of Allied and Professional Bodyworkers (ABMP). Dr. James is also the founder of the first international professional association representing primarily Thai Style bodywork therapist, (International Thai Therapists Association, Inc. ITTA, Inc... now defunct) Having traveled and lived extensively throughout Southeast Asia, he has completed advanced training programs in several different countries i.e. Thailand, Philippines, Indonesia, India and China. His Primary focus, however, is and always has been on the traditional healing arts of Thailand. Dr. James was awarded the prestigious "Friend of Thailand Award" 2002, for development and promotion of Thai classical arts, Thai Massage and Thai Yoga therapies.

On December 1st. 2006, Anantasuk School of Traditional Thai Medicine, Hua Hin Thailand. Dr. Anthony James receives "Aacharn", Master Instructor recognition from the Wat Po Association for Traditional Thai Medicine, Anantasuk School for Traditional Thai Medicine and Wangklaikangwon Industrial Community & Educational College.

Currently Dr. James is directing the day to day development of the NAIC (Native American Indigenous Church, Inc) and the SomaVeda College of Natural Medicine (SCNM): Thai Yoga Center certification program. This 20 to over 4000 hour professional development program consists of five College Degree programs and five Certificate levels and supplemental courses. It is complimentary and designed to have parity with other similar certification courses in traditional religious therapeutics therapies with origins jointly in Ayurveda and Indigenous Native American Medicine. This program, presented nationally and internationally, is setting a high standard at many schools of therapeutic Yoga around the country.

Aachan, Dr. James was a personal apprentice of the 36th GrandMaster Phaa Khruu Samaii Mesamarn of the Buddhai Sawan Institute, Nongkam Thailand. He is a graduate of the Traditional College of Medicine Wat Chetuphon, Bangkok as well as adjunct faculty training program of the Buntautuk Northern Provincial Hospital and Foundation of Shivago Komarpai, Old Medicine Hospital under Aachan Sintorn Chaichagun, Chiangmai Thailand. This book and others authored by Dr. James are currently being used in Thailand to train both Thai and western students. In addition, currently holds Special Faculty Position for several schools in Thailand with formal teaching recognitions from the Royal Thai Departments of Commerce, Trade exports Department and Royal Thai Ministries of Health and Education.

He is recognized formally as a lineage holder and master teacher for several different Indigenous Traditional Thai healing systems including Buddhai Sawan, Buntautuk, Tawee and now through the Wat Po Teachers Association and Union of Thai Traditional Medicine Society as well.

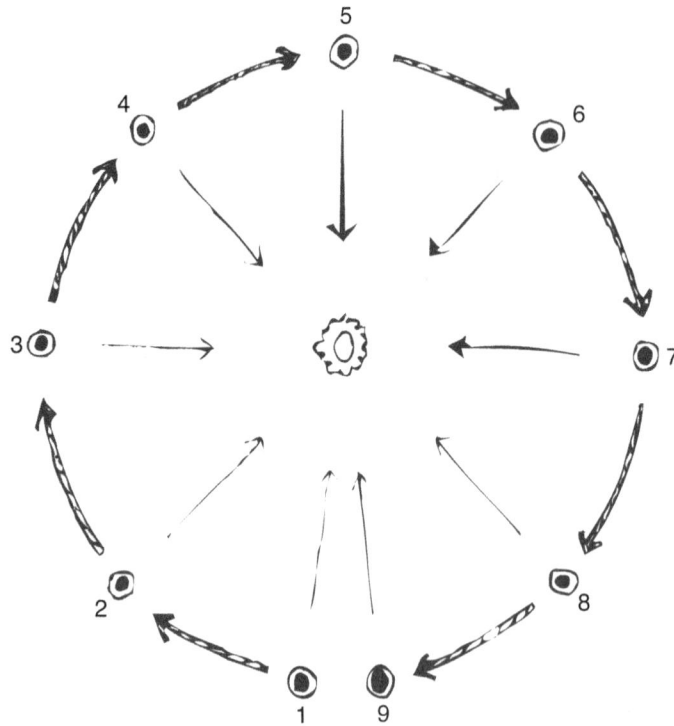

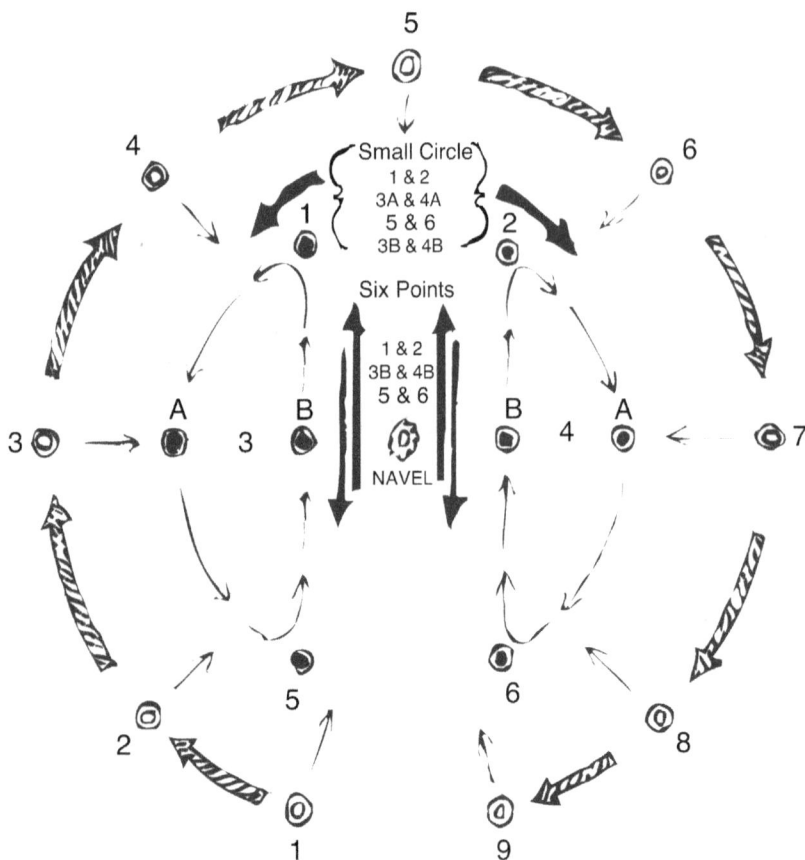

Notes

 Meta Journal Press

Notes

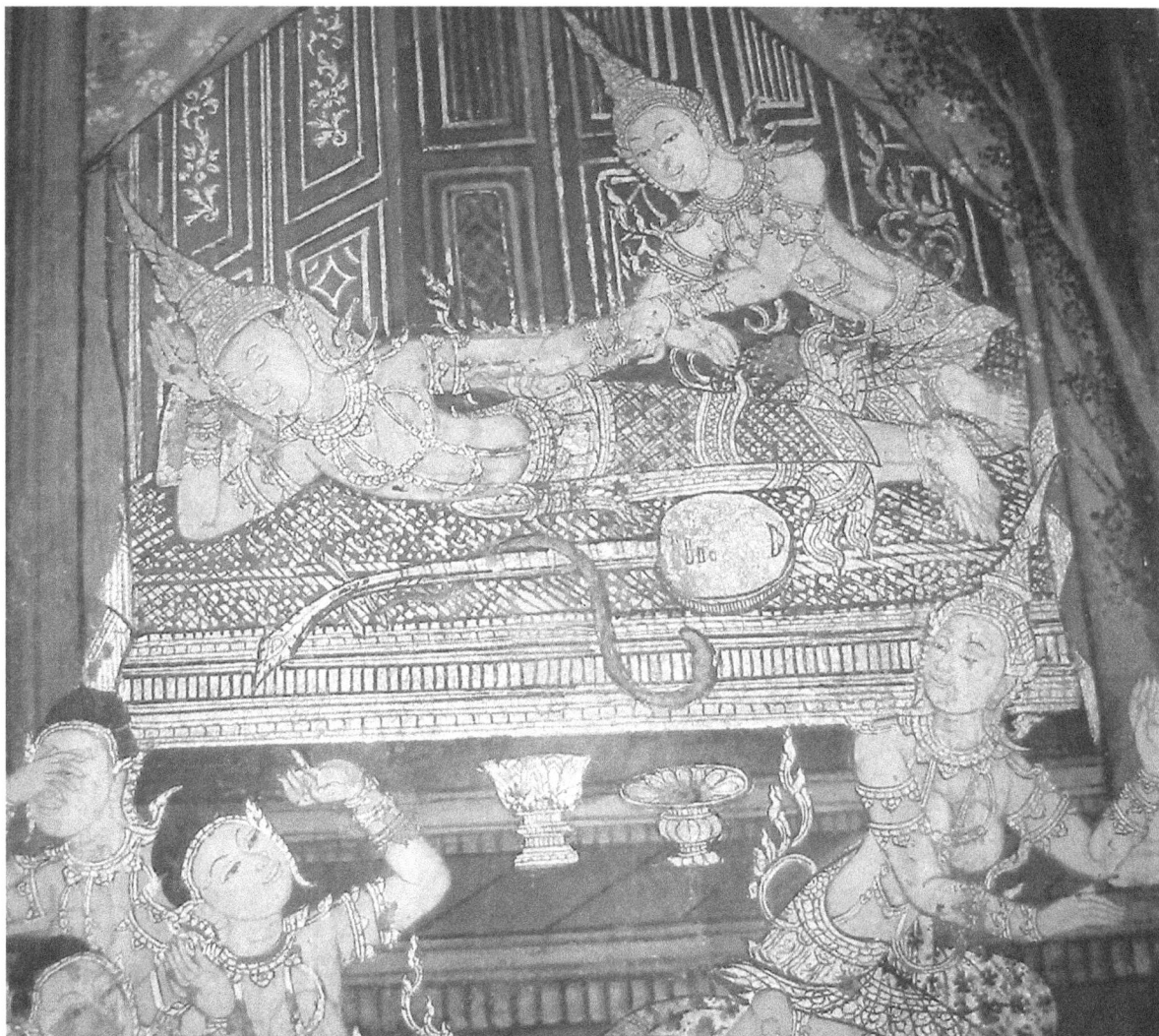

From the Thai Religious Mythology, The Ramayanna, we see the God like King Rama receiving healing Yoga Therapy. Illustration is a photograph taken from the outer courtyard and walls of the Royal Chapel Pavillion, Wat Phra Khaew, Bangkok... considered the most sacred religious shrine in Thai Buddhism. Also known as the Royal Chapel.